D1327520

The Putting Patients First Field Guide

The Putting Patients First Field Guide

Global Lessons in Designing and Implementing Patient-Centered Care

EDITORS

SUSAN B. FRAMPTON

PATRICK A. CHARMEL

SARA GUASTELLO

PLANETREE

JB JOSSEY-BASS™
A Wiley Brand

Cover design: JPuda
Cover image: (map) © sorendls/Getty; (figures) © ImagesbyTrista/istockphoto

Published by Jossey-Bass
A Wiley Brand
One Montgomery Street, Suite 1200, San Francisco, CA 94104-4594—www.josseybass.com

Limit of Liability/Disclaimer of Warranty: While the publisher and author have used their best efforts in
preparing this book, they make no representations or warranties with respect to the accuracy or completeness
of the contents of this book and specifically disclaim any implied warranties of merchantability or fitness for
a particular purpose. No warranty may be created or extended by sales representatives or written sales
materials. The advice and strategies contained herein may not be suitable for your situation. You should
consult with a professional where appropriate. Neither the publisher nor author shall be liable for any loss of
profit or any other commercial damages, including but not limited to special, incidental, consequential, or
other damages. Readers should be aware that Internet Web sites offered as citations and/or sources for
further information may have changed or disappeared between the time this was written and when it is read.

Jossey-Bass books and products are available through most bookstores. To contact Jossey-Bass directly call
our Customer Care Department within the U.S. at 800-956-7739, outside the U.S. at 317-572-3986, or fax
317-572-4002.

Wiley publishes in a variety of print and electronic formats and by print-on-demand. Some material
included with standard print versions of this book may not be included in e-books or in print-on-demand.
If this book refers to media such as a CD or DVD that is not included in the version you purchased, you
may download this material at **http://booksupport.wiley.com**. For more information about Wiley products,
visit **www.wiley.com**.

Library of Congress Cataloging-in-Publication Data
The putting patients first field guide : global lessons in designing and implementing patient-centered care /
editors, Susan B. Frampton, Patrick A. Charmel, Sara Guastello. – First edition.
    p. ; cm.
   Includes bibliographical references and index.
   ISBN 978-1-118-44494-8 (cloth), ISBN 978-1-119-45008-6 (epub), ISBN 978-1-119-45009-3 (ePDF)
   I. Frampton, Susan B., editor of compilation.   II. Charmel, Patrick A., editor of compilation.
III. Guastello, Sara, editor of compilation.
   [DNLM: 1. Patient-Centered Care–methods.   2. Physician-Patient Relations.   3. Quality Assurance,
Health Care–methods. W 84.7]
   R727.3
   610.69'6–dc23
                                         2013011587

Printed in the United States of America

FIRST EDITION

HB Printing   10 9 8 7 6 5 4 3 2 1

CONTENTS

TABLES AND FIGURES

Tables

Figures

This book is dedicated to the continuing inspiration provided to caregivers around the world by the life and work of Laura C. Gilpin (1950–2007).

ACKNOWLEDGMENTS

THIS IS THE third edition of the Putting Patients First series, the first published a decade ago. The success of this series is a testament to the forward-thinking ideas of Planetree's early leaders, led with quiet grace and a strong vision by Angelica Thieriot, who contributed the prologue to this book. These visionaries were defining what it meant to be patient-centered before there was even a term to define. They established a firm foundation for patient-centered care and the Planetree model and philosophy to flourish.

Where it flourishes is in hospitals, medical centers, nursing homes, clinics, physician practices, assisted living communities, behavioral health centers, rehabilitation hospitals, and other care settings where, day in and day out, caregivers devote themselves to the care of others. In putting together this book, we have been humbled by those who have taken on this tremendous responsibility and privilege—often doing so as they try to make the most of scarce resources in the face of many external demands that exert additional pressures. It could be very easy for these caregivers to dismiss patient-centered care as *one more thing to do*, but they don't. Instead, they have approached it as THE thing to do. The ideas and innovations captured throughout these pages originated with them. This book is a testament to their attitudes of compassion and empathy, their resourcefulness, and their creativity.

Our dear friends Laura Gilpin and Harvey Picker embodied these attributes of compassion, empathy, resourcefulness, and creativity. Their spirits and influence are present throughout this book.

Many of the innovations in these pages have originated with health care professionals. Others are examples of codevelopment where patients have gone beyond sharing their experiences with us to guide improvement, and have fully partnered with health care providers to develop and implement practices that improve the health care experience for all involved.

In each edition of this series, it has been a pleasure to invite a diverse group of patient-centered care champions to share their expertise and unique perspectives on what it takes to create and sustain an organizational culture that puts patients first. For this book, as in years past, these requests were consistently met with eager desire to impart knowledge and an enthusiastic willingness to share, despite busy schedules and heavy responsibilities. We are immensely grateful for the time, energy, and effort each contributor dedicated to this project. You will find them listed after The Editors.

In every aspect of creating this book, we have drawn heavily on the experiences of our colleagues around the world from whom we have learned so much. Their support and guidance in this process have been invaluable. We do not have the space to list all of their names, but we wanted to especially thank some key global leaders, including Jim van den Beuken and Marcel Snijders of Planetree Nederland; Lucie Dumas of Réseau Planetree Quebec; Henrique Sutton de Sousa Neves, CEO of Sociedade Beneficente Israelita Brasileira and the staff of Planetree Brazil; Lucile Hanscom of the Picker Institute and Sir Donald Irvine of Picker Europe; Karen Luxford of the Clinical Excellence Commission in Australia; Antonello Zangrandi and Federico Zangrandi of Progea in Italy; Ana Augusta Blumer Salotti; kz Morihiro; Dr. Dorothea Wild; Dr. Etel Veringa; Marie Fuglsang and Karin Jay for being international ambassadors for Planetree, helping to expand patient-centered care around the world and facilitate global sharing of best practices and innovations.

The progress documented in this book builds on the work of many organizations, among them Joint Commission International, the International Society for Quality in Health Care, the National Quality Forum and the National Priorities Partnership, the Picker Institute, the World Health Organization, the Institute for Healthcare Improvement, Health Consumers' Alliance of South Australia, the Saskatchewan Union of Nurses, the Danish Unit of Patient-Perceived Quality, the Arnold P. Gold

Foundation, and the African Patient-Centered Care Initiative led by Peter Arimi of USAID, Fred Wabwire-Magnen of the Regional Centre for Quality in Healthcare and Stephen Kinoti of Fio Corporation.

The Putting Patients First series would not be possible were it not for Andy Pasternack and Seth Schwartz at Jossey-Bass who have been valuable partners on this project. They have guided us through the publishing process, and have worked hard to ensure that the manuscripts we have so painstakingly developed ultimately make it into the hands of readers so that the concepts can be put into practice.

To our draft manuscript reviewers, Karen Adams, Sir Donald Irvine, Jerod M. Loeb, Debra Ness, and Jennifer Sweeney, we thank you for your thoughtful and constructive comments.

We would finally like to acknowledge our colleagues and friends within Planetree—the members of the board of directors and the Planetree International Advisory Council, and an enormously talented staff for whom patient-centered care is nothing less than a personal mission. It is an honor to work with this brilliant group of people as we turn the page to Planetree's next chapter.

Susan B. Frampton, Patrick A. Charmel, and Sara Guastello
The Editors

SUSAN B. FRAMPTON, PHD

For over a decade, Dr. Susan Frampton has been the president of Planetree, a nonprofit advocacy, consultation, and membership organization that works with a growing network of hospitals and continuing care communities around the world to implement Planetree's comprehensive patient- and person-centered model of care. Dr. Frampton has authored numerous publications, the most recent including a series on patient-centered care in the *American Journal of Nursing, International Health Federation Journal, Patient-Centered Care Improvement Guide, Long-Term Care Improvement Guide*, and the edited collection *Putting Patients First*, Second Edition (Jossey-Bass, 2008). The first edition of *Putting Patients First* (Jossey-Bass, 2003) won the ACHE Hamilton Book of the Year Award in 2004.

In 2013, Dr. Frampton was appointed cochair of the National Priorities Partnership (NPP), a collaborative of fifty-two major national organizations working to identify strategies for improving safety, quality, and patient-centered outcomes for the U.S. health care system. Her work with the National Priorities Partnership extends back to 2009, when she was first named a member. In 2011, she served on NPP's Better Care Subcommittee, which helped to shape a set of comprehensive national goals to improve the quality of health and health care. She also was cochair of the NPP (Re)admissions Action Team, which developed and executed strategies to safely reduce avoidable readmissions and increase the uptake of patient-centered team-based care delivery models. In addition to this work with NPP, Dr. Frampton has participated on the Joint Commission's Expert Advisory Panel on culturally competent patient-centered care standards, the National Quality Forum's Care Coordination Steering Team and the Institute of Medicine's review panel for their 2009 publication on integrative medicine.

In addition to speaking internationally on culture change, quality and safety, and the patient experience, she has presented keynotes on designing patient-centered practices in acute care, continuing care, and ambulatory medicine settings for various hospital associations, Veterans Health Administration, and the World Health Organization. In addition, Dr. Frampton was honored in 2009, when she was named one of "20 People Who Make Healthcare Better" by *Health Leaders Magazine*.

PATRICK A. CHARMEL, MPH, FACHE

Patrick A. Charmel, president and chief executive officer of Griffin Hospital and its parent organization, Griffin Health Services Corporation, has been associated with Griffin since 1979, when he served as a student intern while attending Quinnipiac University. He became president in 1998. As president of Griffin Health Services Corporation, he is also the chief executive officer of Planetree Inc., a subsidiary corporation. Under his leadership, Griffin has appeared on the *Fortune* magazine list of the 100 Best Companies to Work for in America for ten consecutive years. The Griffin Hospital management team was selected as the 2008 Top Leadership Team in Healthcare in the nation for community and mid-size hospitals by HealthLeaders Media. Griffin has been the recipient of numerous quality, value, and patient experience awards from various national organizations that measure and monitor hospital performance. Griffin is the only Connecticut hospital named a Top Quality Performer by The Joint Commission, the leading accreditor of health care organizations in America. Griffin Hospital was also recognized by the Premier healthcare alliance as a winner of the 2010 Premier Award for Quality, putting it in the top 1 percent of the nation's hospitals. Griffin also received this award in 2007.

Charmel is a coeditor of the book *Putting Patients First*, which received the American College of Healthcare Executive's Health Care Book of the Year award in 2004. A second edition of the book was released in October 2008.

In 2008, he completed a three-year term as a member of the National Advisory Council for Healthcare Research and Quality, to which he was appointed by the U.S. Secretary for Health and Human Services. He also serves as immediate past chairman of the board of directors of the Connecticut Hospital Association, formerly served as chairman of the Greater Valley Chamber of Commerce board of directors, and currently serves as chairman of the board of Diversified Network Service (DNS), the Connecticut Hospital Association's for-profit subsidiary.

Charmel is the immediate past chairman of the board of governors of the Quinnipiac University Alumni Association and a former university trustee. Quinnipiac University honored him with the Distinguished Alumni Award in 2008. In 2011, he received the Distinguished Alumni Award from the Yale School of Public Health. In 2006 he was the recipient of the John D. Thompson Distinguished Visiting Fellow Award at Yale University. He is a recipient of the James E. West Fellow Award from the Boy Scouts of America and the 2009 Planetree Lifetime Achievement Award.

SARA GUASTELLO

Sara Guastello is director of Knowledge Management for Planetree. In this role, she oversees the Patient-Centered Hospital Designation Program and the associated Patient-Centered Merit Recognition Program, the only such program to recognize excellence in person-centered care across the continuum of care and around the world. Sara collaborates and consults with Planetree members and other partners to heighten awareness and understanding of patient- and person-centered approaches to care. She has authored numerous publications, including articles in the *American Journal of Nursing* Patients First Series, the *International Hospital Federation World Hospitals and Health Services Journal*, *Provider* magazine, *The Patient* journal, and *Food Studies: An Interdisciplinary Journal*. She has authored white papers on integrating the patient and family voice into hospital operations and advancing person-centered care across the continuum, and developed a series of toolkits spotlighting field-tested strategies for

HCAHPS improvement. With support from The Picker Institute, she led the efforts to create the *Patient-Centered Care Improvement Guide* and the companion *Long-Term Care Improvement Guide*, comprehensive compendiums of premier patient- and resident-centered practices in place at health care organizations around the world.

THE CONTRIBUTORS

Róisín Boland, RGN, MBA, former chief executive officer, International Society for Quality in Health Care

Michelle Bowman, BSN, RN, LAc, nursing director, Longmont United Hospital, Longmont, Colorado

Randall L. Carter, senior vice president, Planetree

Catherine Crock, MD, executive director, Australian Institute for Patient and Family Centred Care; physician, Royal Children's Hospital, Melbourne, Australia

Belinda Dewar, PhD, MSc, RGN, RCNT, professor of practice improvement, Institute of Care and Practice Improvement, University of West Scotland, Hamilton, Scotland, UK

Sylvie Doiron, clinical services director, Centre de réadaptation Estrie, Sherbrooke, Quebec

Sir Liam Donaldson, chair in health policy, Imperial College, London; World Health Organization Patient Safety Envoy

Lucie Dumas, CEO, Centre de réadaptation Estrie, Sherbrooke, Quebec; CEO and founder, Réseau Planetree Quebec

Deborah Felsenthal, manager of patients, families and consumers center, Patient-Centered Primary Care Collaborative

John T. Findley, MD, Planetree physician consultant, Valley View Hospital, Glenwood Springs, Colorado

José Henrique Germann Ferreira, MD, CEO, Management Consultancy, Albert Einstein Hospital, São Paulo, Brazil

Richard E. Hanke, EdD, SPHR, leadership development & coaching consultant; founding co-chair, Patient Partnership Council, Delnor Hospital, Geneva, Illinois

Steven F. Horowitz, MD, FACC, medical director, Planetree and Cardiac Care Management, Stamford Hospital, Stamford, Connecticut; professor of clinical medicine, Columbia University College of Physicians and Surgeons, New York; Physician Liaison, Planetree

Edward Kelley, PhD, executive coordinator, WHO Patient Safety Programme

Joep P. Koch, MBA-Health Care, Sector Manager Treatment, Planetree coordinator, Rivas Zorggroep, Gorinchem, The Netherlands

Anna Lee, programme officer, Patients for Patient Safety, WHO

K. J. Lee, MD, FACS, associate clinical professor, Yale University; emeritus chief of otolaryngology, Hospital of St. Raphael, New Haven, Connecticut

Claudio Luiz Lottenberg, president, Sociedade Beneficente Israelita Brasileira Hospital Albert Einstein, São Paulo, Brazil

Karen Luxford, PhD, FAIM, FAAQHC, director, Patient Based Care, Clinical Excellence Commission, Sydney, Australia

Jeanette Michalak, RN, MSN, vice president, Clinical Services, Planetree

Marci Nielsen, PhD, MPH, chief executive officer, Patient-Centered Primary Care Collaborative

Dennis S. O'Leary, MD, president emeritus, The Joint Commission

Anna W. J. Omtzigt, MD, PhD, chairman, medical board, Flevo Hospital, Almere, The Netherlands; medical director, Vrouw & Klinieken, The Netherlands

Dan Otero, BSHA, CLP, LSSBB senior coach, Patient-Centered Lean

Lisa Platt, RID, LEED AP BD+C, EDAC, Planetree consultation service specialist

Marie-Claude Poulin, Planetree coordinator and communications officer, Centre de réadaptation Estrie, Sherbrooke, Quebec; consultant, Réseau Planetree Quebec

Nittita Prasopa-Plaizier, MPH, MHSc, programme manager and technical lead, Patients for Patient Safety Programme, World Health Organization

Heidi Ruis, area manager integrated care, Rivas Zorggroep, Gorinchem, The Netherlands

Marcel Snijders, founder/board member; Designation Specialist, Planetree Nederland

Susan Stone, PhD, RN, NEA-BC, senior vice president and CEO, Sharp Coronado Hospital and Healthcare Center, Coronado, California

Angelica Thieriot, founder, Planetree

Jim van den Beuken, founder and chairman, Planetree Nederland; managing partner, Creative Power

Dorothea Wild, MD, MPH, dr. med., president, Griffin Faculty Practice Plan; associate program director, Combined Internal Medicine and Preventive Medicine Residency Program, Griffin Hospital, Derby, Connecticut

Paula Wilson, president and chief executive officer, Joint Commission Resources/Joint Commission International

PROLOGUE

THIRTY-FIVE YEARS AGO I was hospitalized with a mysterious virus. What I encountered at the hospital was both surprising and devastating.

Soon after arriving I, in essence, lost my citizenship to the human race. I was no longer an adult with rights and privileges.

My privacy, my modesty, my autonomy, and my identity were taken from me when I was most vulnerable—desperately ill and afraid.

As I slumped in a wheelchair behind six or seven other patients (an accurate if unfortunate word to describe a person in a hospital) also slumping in a badly lit basement hallway awaiting X-rays, I became certain that I wouldn't make it out of that place alive.

The window in my room faced a light well. It was impossible to tell in that penumbra if it was sunny or cloudy, or what time of day it was. There were medical artifacts in my room and all manner of things beeping. The only recognizable object in the room was a chair in the corner.

Every morning I was awakened at dawn (having just fallen asleep a couple of hours before) with an extravagantly unsuitable breakfast.

Each nurse was a new, rushed face, nobody could answer my questions, nobody knew my name. I was prodded and poked with no explanation. "Ask your doctor" was all I was ever told.

The doctor talked to my husband about me as if I wasn't there, at one point saying, "I'm afraid we are losing her."

Six years before I had moved up to California from Buenos Aires, Argentina, where I was born. While I lived there I gave birth to two children in local hospitals. Those hospitals had normal furniture, curtains, rugs, wall art, and flowers. The nurses were warm and attentive, the food was good, and I felt cared for and safe. Granted I was not ill, but the same hospital was caring for all kinds of patients in the same way. Perhaps the technology was not up to U.S. standards but the experience was much more humane and healing. We knew then, as now, that stress and fear are obstacles to healing. What could be more stressful than to lose your identity and all control over your life and your person?

My virus was self-limiting and after three weeks in the hospital I went home determined to either change the way American hospitals worked, or return to South America—making sure that if I should fall ill again I would never have to endure that experience again.

The next six months were spent thinking about what I would have wanted during my illness—what I NEEDED to get better.

During that period I researched the history of hospitals, and found out that, in the West, the only glorious period for hospitals was the Hellenic. The asclepian hospitals (dedicated to the god of healing, Asclepius) were set in the most beautiful places, by sacred groves. They used art, theater, music, and poetry to revitalize the patient's healing energies and acceded to their subconscious with ritual acts and dream incubation. Patients were given herbal potions and instructed to go to the "abaton" and dream of their healing, which they did to good effect. They used nutrition and herbal medicines and kept really good records which we have to this day. Guess what: it worked!

Thankfully, we now also have extraordinary medicines and miraculous surgeries. So why not have them be administered in the best healing environments possible?

As I dreamed of my ideal healing place I thought first about the human environment, and how I would have loved a calm focused presence to reassure me.

Nurses go into their profession from a deep desire to heal, to make people feel better, safe, comfortable, and free of pain. It is too demanding and selfless a career to embark upon without a deep altruistic calling.

The difference between the Argentine and American nurses of the 1980s was that the systems that the United States had developed to adapt to high volume and technology had not taken human values into account. I fear that as hospitals modernize around the world they are replicating some of these efficiencies that are so dehumanizing and eventually inefficient.

Wards had (have?) acuity ratings within which nurses were deployed, like widgets, according to a score determined by how ill the patients were. That's why I never saw the same nurse twice. What was needed, I realized, was primary care nursing, each nurse getting a number of patients for whom he or she is responsible. That's how nursing worked in less technologically advanced parts of the world. And that's how nurses get to feel they are truly healing people, how they see the outcome of their care.

Also I thought that nurses needed to be reminded of their calling periodically—and be nurtured and supported to allow them to encounter so much suffering without losing themselves. The person who developed deep ways to do this was Laura Gilpin, our "First Nurse." When we first interviewed her she said, "I like making it safe for my patients to sleep." That's the nurse I was looking for!

What I needed most of all was to feel seen and respected, to have the sense that someone cared about my well-being and that my needs would be met. I needed to retain some control, to be informed, in ways I could understand, about what tests were going to be performed, which procedures and why.

One of the first members of the original Planetree board, prominent San Francisco doctor John Gamble, had started a project called PIIR node—patients informed, involved, and responsible. Although this project succumbed to internal hospital politics, it nevertheless provided many useful examples of ways to educate and inform.

Our first director, Ryan Phelan, came from a public resource and information background. In addition to her brilliant ability to turn ideas into working programs, her particular interest in empowering patients by providing them with access to high-quality information was key to the success of our first resource centers and the development of educational materials for hospitalized patients. In the days before the Internet this was an even more unique and valuable resource.

It struck me as odd that we put enormous amounts of effort and money into beautifying airports, hotel lobbies, restaurants, offices, not to mention our own homes, while neglecting the environments within which we spend some of the most important moments of our lives—our own birth, life-changing illnesses, surgeries, and our death as well as these events in the lives of our loved ones—moments of openness, when all our assumptions about our life are up for review; these are eminently teachable moments.

Many studies have shown the impact of the physical environment on healing. From the need for pain medications to length of stay, just being able to look at a tree from the window has an important, measurable impact.

When I went from the daydreaming phase to talking to real people in the field I met architect Roslyn Lindheim, who had dedicated a large part of her career to creating humanized hospital settings. Before we opened our first model unit, she had herself admitted as a patient for two days to see what was needed. The effect of light, color, clutter, sound, beauty, art, doorways, hallways, privacy, the accessibility of the nursing staff—she encountered all of these issues, and with the help of designer Victoria Fay came up with creative and beautiful environments that support healing.

To this day I feel Planetree is evolving new solutions, new ways of adapting to different cultural cues and changing perceptions of beauty and comfort. Wonderful designers and architects have found new ways of improving the environments of hospitals.

I wanted my family and my close friends around me, mainly for support and companionship, but also to bring me food I could eat. I learned that many elderly patients were suffering from malnutrition because they couldn't eat hospital food. It became obvious that with the variety of cultures represented in any patient population, the only way to deal with food preferences and needs was to provide a kitchenette for families to prepare meals.

Also the rising costs of care make it hard to improve the quality of the food provided by the hospital, although I still dream of the hospital as a place to teach patients and families about nutrition and healthy eating. (Years after the beginning of Planetree, I sat with my husband, who was having a heart attack in a cardiac intensive care ward, and watched a breakfast of scrambled eggs, bacon, and coffee delivered to his bedside. (Fortunately he survived.)

The wonderful thing about the modern world is that (possibly thanks to the Internet) people are now empowered to make informed decisions in all aspects of life. We should all claim that right and that privilege, especially when it comes to our health and survival.

Many cultures from around the world have developed ancient modes of healing that work every bit as well as ours. (I myself have seen the symptoms of my Parkinson's disease hugely improved by Chinese mushroom supplements.) Traditional practices should be made available to hospital patients in their own countries as well as in the United States. Modernizing should not exclude traditional modalities that are safe and healing.

Because Planetree has a life of its own and draws the right people to further its goals, it continues to grow and evolve and incorporate new research into the nature of healing environments.

As the retired grandmother of Planetree, I am always thrilled and delighted to see all the new ways in which Planetree has developed.

As a patient I rebelled against being denied my humanity, and that rebellion led to the beginnings of Planetree. We should all demand to be treated as competent adults, and take an active part in our healing. And we should insist on hospitals meeting our human need for respect, control, warm and supportive care, a harmonious environment, and good, healthy food. A truly healing environment.

Angelica Thieriot

DIGNITY, RESPECT, COMPASSION, answering difficult questions, asking someone to say back what they have heard, smiling, expressing empathy without losing objectivity. Traditionally, these and other profound human skills have been little taught or discussed at medical and nursing schools. Indeed, there are many senior doctors who believe that they cannot be taught. Even worse, some view them as peripheral concerns when the real business is understanding why the body-machine is malfunctioning and finding ways to correct it.

It is not that patients do not want the science, technology, and rational clinical assessment and intervention, but they also want the deep connection to them as a person. People with cancer surely want the best chance of survival that modern medicine can offer them, but they also need someone to listen, understand, and explain. They want someone to show solidarity with a fellow human being who is suffering. They want to be the owner of their care, not just a by-product of it.

This challenge is not only for practitioners; it is for those who manage health organizations and for those who lead health care systems. To know that your system is as safe as it can be and to be sure that every single episode of care is truly patient-centered is a formidable task. Yet this should not be the stuff of aspirations; it must be the very fabric of concrete, measurable delivery of care.

What is particularly inspiring about this book is the wealth of practical examples, experiences, and stories from the front line of care by patients, family members, and practitioners.

For anyone who has experienced care personally or through a loved one, there are many things in the chapters that resonate powerfully. Among a telling list of negative interactions with older people in one example in the book is "using childlike language or elder-speak." How many times has a baby boomer son or daughter felt anger, disbelief, and despair at hearing their elderly mother or father spoken to that way in a hospital, particularly if their communication is impaired (say, through a stroke)?

The Berlin Wall of traditional health care, where it remains, must come down. The philosophy of care set out in this book is not a technocratic matter to sit in a health system's strategic plan. It is the foundation on which a modern health system should be built. Without it, the morality and humanity of care will crumble.

Planetree is an organization that has pioneered the modern movement of patient-centered care. Their work is a touchstone for a new world when the vision becomes a reality, not just in islands of excellence but in the whole land-mass of health care.

This book opens the door of opportunity for all health care providers to be inspired to transform their organizations.

Sir Liam Donaldson
chair in health policy, Imperial College, London
World Health Organization Patient Safety Envoy

The Putting Patients First Field Guide

Introduction
Patient-Centered Care Goes Global

L ISTENING AND CARING. Compassion and comfort. Humanity and respect. Partnership and engagement. The themes at the heart of patient-centered care date back to the origins of modern medicine. Hippocrates is quoted as teaching the earliest medical students, "Treat often, cure sometimes, comfort always." About the significance of the role of nurses, nursing pioneer Florence Nightingale wrote, "[Nursing] has been limited to signify little more than the administration of medicines and the application of poultices. It ought to signify the proper use of fresh air, light, warmth, cleanliness, quiet and the proper selection and administration of diet—all at the least expense of vital power to the patient" (1860). Nearly seventy years later Francis Peabody, MD, a renowned physician who fell terminally ill, shared his insights on caregiving: "The treatment of a disease may be entirely impersonal; the care of a patient must be completely personal" and "The secret of the care of the patient is in caring for the patient" (1927).

This Introduction is based on interviews with Lucie Dumas, founder, Réseau Planetree Quebec; José Henrique Germann Ferreira, MD, CEO, management consultancy, Hospital Israelita Albert Einstein, Brazil; Susan B. Frampton, PhD, president, Planetree; Dr. Claudio Luiz Lottenberg, president, Sociedade Beneficiente Israelita Brasileira Albert Einstein, Brazil; Karen Luxford, director, Patient Based Care, Clinical Excellence Commission, Australia; and Jim van den Beuken, founder and chairman, Planetree Nederland.

PATIENT-CENTERED CARE: A CRESTING WAVE OF CHANGE

There is nothing about patient-centered care (or patient-based, person-centered, client-centered, or relationship-centered care) that is cutting edge. And yet, while the concept is truly timeless, it is also especially timely. This book is the third installment of the Putting Patients First series. The first was published a decade ago. At that time, patient-centered care was just beginning to gain traction as the optimal way to deliver care, fueled in large part by a landmark Institute of Medicine study that identified patient-centeredness as one of six primary determinants of health care quality and defined it as: "Health care that establishes a partnership among practitioners, patients and their families (when appropriate) to ensure that decisions respect patients' wants, needs, and preferences and that patients have the education and support they require to make decisions and participate in their own care" (Institute of Medicine, 2001).

In the wake of this high-profile endorsement, efforts to expand patient-centered care have been slow but steady, propelled largely by individual champions and their powerful stories of person-centeredness in action. Today, though, in countries around the world, there is a cresting wave of interest in patient-centered care, driven by powerful industry forces, a growing evidence base, and the demands of increasingly discerning health care consumers.

A Changing Global Health Care Landscape

Since the publication of the first *Putting Patients First* book, the global health care landscape has shifted. Consumers have ready access to an unprecedented amount of data on diseases, treatments, and health care providers. They are connecting on blogs and social media sites with others who share similar conditions, logging on to online personal health portals, using search engines to guide self-directed health research, and downloading apps for their smartphones to help manage their health. Unquestionably, patients as a whole are more informed than ever before when they meet with their care providers. As a result, they increasingly expect to be engaged in a dialogue about their diagnosis, treatment options, and personal health goals, and to contribute in a meaningful way to the care planning process.

Consumers today not only have access to more information about medical conditions and treatment options, but also about providers. Public ratings and rank-ordered lists of health centers along with quality accreditations are becoming common in many countries. Greater transparency in the sharing of quality and patient experience outcomes and new governmental incentives to publicly report them equip today's consumers with an array of qualitative and quantitative data to inform their decisions of where to go for care.

Consumers have come to expect an abundance of choices in virtually every major (and not-so-major) purchase that they make. Why would health care be an exception—especially now when out-of-pocket health care expenses continue to rise? To remain competitive, health care organizations must be responsive to the full range of patient needs, preferences, and values, and be prepared to withstand the scrutiny and informed decision making of today's health care purchasers, be they individuals, employers, or governments.

The medical tourism industry takes the concept of choice to a new level and is compelling health care providers around the world to seek out ways to differentiate themselves in order to attract patients and revenue from outside their local regions.

At the same time, we are experiencing a global demographic shift. An aging population requires already overburdened, underfunded health care systems to meet the demands of increasingly vulnerable patients contending with chronic diseases, multiple morbidities, and cognitive impairments. Efficient and effective use of resources to optimize outcomes requires that care be coordinated across the full continuum of services and be organized around the person, versus around a discrete episode of care or a specific care setting.

Global Health Care Reform Efforts Promote Patient-Centered Care

All of these factors have created conditions in which patient-centered care stands to flourish. Indeed, around the world, health care delivery systems are undergoing reforms to improve outcomes and maximize value. Field experience and research corroborate that engaging with patients and their family members, welcoming their involvement as integral members of the care team, and supporting health care professionals to forge these partnerships establishes the foundation for superior outcomes, fewer errors, lower readmissions, and high patient and family satisfaction. As a result, patient-centered care is consistently being identified as a fundamental strategy of these reform efforts for achieving high-quality, high-value care. Gone are the days when patient-centered care could be dismissed as something that is "nice" to do should resources allow. Today, patient-centered care is nothing less than a quality and business imperative.

A quick scan of reform efforts currently under way around the world reveals that there are numerous avenues for advancing the adoption of patient-centered care, and many levers for promoting this change.

- Brazil's National Policy of Humanization, adopted in 2003, emphasizes the importance of listening and dialogue to the establishment of caring, humanistic relationships between patients and professional caregivers. Today, the policy is redefining what it means to provide quality care, and is driving significant transformation in the culture of health care in that country.

- A continent away, the African Patient-Centered Care Initiative (APCCI) Task Force has embarked on the development of an African patient-centered health care model, providing leadership and advocacy to advance application of the model throughout sub-Saharan Africa. This effort is supported by The Regional Centre for Quality Health Care (RCQHC), The United States Agency for International Development (USAID), and key stakeholders including representatives from regional hospitals and university health centers, patient representative groups, Health Ministries, and the World Health Organization.

- In Australia, new national health care accreditation standards heavily emphasize consumer partnership, with one of the ten standards devoted entirely to partnerships with consumers in governance. To support health care professionals in complying with the new standards, the accrediting body is releasing a range of guides on strategies for partnering with consumers. In New South Wales, the Clinical Excellence Commission has issued *The Patient Based Care Challenge* to all public sector health district boards. The Challenge encourages governance to implement patient-based approaches as part of the longer-term strategic goals of the organization. Examples include promoting consumer engagement in board or safety and quality committees, actively using patient feedback to drive change and implementing patient- and family-activated escalation (or patient- and family-activated rapid response teams) for deteriorating patients.

- In the United States, hospitals' performance on the nationally standardized Hospital Consumer Assessment of Healthcare Providers and Systems (HCAHPS) patient experience survey is dictating a portion of their federal reimbursement payments, for the first time explicitly tying reimbursement levels to the quality of the patient experience. In the spirit of organizing care around the patient, the establishment of accountable care organizations (local networks of providers that manage the full continuum of care for all patients within their provider network) is a centerpiece of the strategy for reforming the U.S. health care system. The government has also incorporated numerous person-centered care principles and language into its regulatory guidelines for nursing homes. These efforts seek to better balance safety and quality of life.

- In Quebec, the Ministry of Health and Social Services has issued a directive aimed at increasing employee recruitment and retention, with all network establishments required to initiate one of three preapproved approaches by early 2015. Recognizing the interconnectivity between the patient experience and the staff experience, among the three approaches is implementation of the Planetree model of patient-centered care.

- Even in the Netherlands, which arguably has one of the world's best health care systems, the forces of health care consumerism are fueling a push toward transparency of quality data and heightened efforts among organizations to differentiate themselves as providers of not only safe and competent care, but also compassionate, person-centered care. The adoption of the CQI Index as a standardized measure of the patient experience is supporting Dutch patients in making more informed decisions about where they receive their care.

More broadly, the creation of patient rights charters and the rise in prominence and influence of patient advocacy groups are amplifying the voices of health care consumers to ensure that international, regional, and national health care policies reflect patients' priorities.

The good news is that in industrialized and developing nations, the efforts to advance patient-centered care are growing stronger and more diversified. Numerous policy, funding, accreditation, public reporting, and business levers are shifting the orientation of health care delivery systems from being provider-centered and setting-centered to being person-centered.

At a national and state level, there has been an increasing recognition of patient-centred approaches in the safety and quality agenda as a key domain of quality care. This is typified by the establishment of my own role as Director of Patient Based Care at the Clinical Excellence Commission (a safety and quality agency) in New South Wales. . . . The only way is up! When you get contacted by specialist

doctors wanting to start Facebook pages for their patients to post direct feedback you know things are starting to move!
—**Karen Luxford, director, Patient Based Care, Clinical Excellence Commission, Australia**

STILL MUCH WORK TO BE DONE

Nonetheless, as a global community of health care providers, we have much work to do to realize this vision of patient-centered care as the norm, versus the exception, in health care. Indeed, emerging industry forces present both challenges and opportunities for spreading person-centered care.

Provider-Centered Care Remains the Norm

Despite recent progress toward greater patient-centeredness, around the world health care remains largely provider-centered. This is in no way a condemnation of the committed individuals who enter the health care profession, most of whom are working hard to provide the best care they can within the constraints imposed by well-established provider-centric traditions. The customary practice of turning on bright overhead lights in a patient room in the middle of the night to check the patient's vital signs comes to mind. Another classic example is the time-honored open-backed hospital gown, which although practical for providers delivering hands-on care, can feel undignified for those wearing them. Participation in these distinctly provider-centered practices is not a reflection of individual care-givers' disregard for people's feelings, but rather a reflection of systems organized around the convenience of providers. This is why patient-centered care, though not rocket science, is far from a quick fix. Delivering care in a person-centered manner is less about modifying specific provider-centric practices, and more about transforming systems, attitudes, and behaviors. It is about culture change.

An important aspect to implementing patient-centered care is related to the need for change in management style. The management style with a tendency toward centralization, bureaucratization, and vertical orientation causes work to occur independently and in isolation, valuing interests and objectives without considering the vision of the organization as a whole and without prioritizing the needs of patients and families. Open communication and respect for the right of expression of users, caregivers, and managers allows a discussion on the differences and limitations of services, the participation of all in decision making and the construction of a new model.

—**José Henrique Germann Ferreira, MD, CEO, management consultancy, Hospital Israelita Albert Einstein, and Dr. Claudio Luiz Lottenberg, president, Sociedade Beneficiente Israelita Brasileira Albert Einstein**

Breaking Down Silos

An essential component of this culture change work must be to synchronize disconnected silos of care so that they can work effectively together around the person at the center. This challenge is hardly unique to any one country or health delivery model. A 2011 survey found that gaps in care coordination, transitions between hospitals and other community-based settings, lapses in communication between specialists and primary care physicians, failure to review medications, and delays in receiving test results were present in all of the eleven industrialized countries examined (Schoen and others, 2011). Reorganizing care around the person at the center is a viable solution for breaking down these silos and addressing these well-documented gaps in care.

Connecting the Dots Between Patient-Centered Care and Quality

There is a strong fragmented approach on patient-centered care where safety is seen as a medical responsibility and hospitality and experience as patient-centered care. We believe that integrating safe, competent, and compassionate care for the human experience—patients, families, and caregivers—matters and makes a big difference.

**—Jim van den Beuken, founder and chairman,
Planetree Nederland**

Another challenge that prevents adoption of person-centered care more broadly is a disjointed way of thinking that segregates out patient-centered care from the more technical and traditional realms of quality and safety. Around the world, the main focus for health care performance continues to be on technical care, clinical outcomes, and financial viability, with less regard for the patient experience. Given the degree to which all these aspects of care are intertwined, we know that there are many opportunities to transform traditionally excellent clinical care into truly exceptional patient-centered care. Organizations must closely examine the patient experience as a critical component of the quality equation.

Compassion First

Advances in policy, health care consumerism, and technology are occurring against the backdrop of a global recession. As health care organizations struggle to maintain a healthy bottom line, they are seeking out ways to deliver safe care as efficiently as possible. Unfortunately, in a growing trend, the casualties of this balancing act are too often compassion, dignity, kindness, and respect.

As just one example, in the wake of revelations about deplorable care provided to patients within the United Kingdom's National Health Service (NHS), public officials have called for changes to restore compassion to the NHS. In a 2012 speech, Health Secretary Jeremy Hunt denounced that "in places that should be devoted to patients, where compassion should be uppermost, we find its very opposite: a coldness, resentment, indifference, even contempt" (Adams, 2012).

As expressed by Mary, who received care in a large hospital in Sydney, Australia, "I could not fault the technical care. However, I was treated like a lump of clay. People came and went from my room, did things to me and no one even spoke to me." Mary is not faulting the hospital from a clinical standpoint, nor is she even criticizing the hospital for failing to provide amenities, hospitality, or customer service (each often mistakenly equated to patient-centeredness). For Mary, the shortcoming of her patient experience was its lack of humanity, kindness, and warmth. Through the lens of quality and safety, where this hospital fell short was in creating a foundation of trust and actively engaging Mary as a member of her own care team.

> It is important to understand the healing power of the emotional connection between patients and their caregivers. The evidence base linking empathy on the part of clinicians and better patient outcomes truly makes kindness and compassion a health care quality imperative.
>
> **—Susan B. Frampton, president, Planetree**

As will be further explored in Chapter Three, compassion is a fundamental element of patient-centeredness. Cold, impersonal care cannot be patient-centered as it fails to honor the humanity of the person at the center. The introduction of new health care policies, quality mandates, reimbursement incentives, and person-centered accreditation standards will be abject failures if we do not first and foremost ground all of this work in an expectation of basic human kindness, dignity, and respect. This requires that we examine what factors in our health care systems are compelling decent, honorable individuals who make their living taking care of others to provide care that is lacking in compassion.

> The increase in membership of Réseau Planetree Quebec is an indicator of this growing interest [in patient-centered care]. One of the

factors that contributes to this increase: acknowledgment of the limits of our health care system regarding its capacity to respond to human needs.

—**Lucie Dumas, founder, Réseau Planetree Quebec**

THE PATIENT EXPERIENCE IS THE HUMAN EXPERIENCE

This third installment of the Putting Patients First series reflects the growing global emphasis on patient-centered care. It incorporates the experiences of health care professionals from more than a dozen countries on six continents. This diversity of experiences has made for a rich study of what it takes to deliver patient-centered care in the context of different health care delivery systems, regulatory environments, payment models, and cultural expectations. What stands out far more profoundly than these differences, however, is the universality of what patients, their loved ones, and their professional caregivers all over the world deem most important about their health care experiences.

What Do Patients Want?

Examining the answer to this question is the focus of the Planetree organization. Following the experience she detailed in the prologue to this book, Angelica Thieriot, along with a small but mighty board of directors, founded Planetree in 1978 as a not-for-profit organization. Planetree vowed to evaluate the totality of the health care experience from the patient's perspective. The organization has long recognized that understanding the patient perspective is only part of what it takes to deliver person-centered care. Changing health care culture to put patients first will only occur when leaders allocating resources and staff at the point of care are actively engaged with patients in the redesign of systems and processes. To this end, over the past three decades, Planetree has facilitated thousands of focus groups with individuals who interact with the health care system in a variety of capacities, asking what matters most to them about their health care experiences, and if they were making the rules, what they would change about the current way hospitals, long-term care communities, and other care settings operate.

While the concepts of person-centered care shape the patient experience at a deeply personal level, these focus groups have underscored the commonalities of the human experience as it relates to health care. The dialogues have yielded remarkably consistent themes that transcend cultures and geographic borders. In general, most patients feel confident that they will receive competent technical care when they enter a hospital or health care center. Beyond that, what matters most to them is being treated with kindness, compassion, and dignity.

> "I think nurses and doctors know their jobs so well that they forget that you don't. So even though they explain it, maybe the warmth isn't there because you don't know what to expect. Like 'you're going to get a pinch.' Well, what next? Maybe just a little more compassion."

Patients want information, choices, and open communication.

> "I always want to participate in my health care, and I think they think I ask too many questions. It seems like I need to get through them just to keep them on their tight schedule."

They want their care to be coordinated. They want their professional caregivers to recognize and embrace the indispensable role that their families, *however they define the term*, play in their care and healing.

> "At some point, [my husband] had a test result and they didn't know why and I knew it to be a reaction to medication. . . . I've taken care of him for ten years with his Parkinson's and I know a lot and she didn't want to listen to me. She put him through two spinal taps and at that point, I said, 'No.' . . . How dare she say that I am hysterical. Of course I am! The person I love is in a very bad situation."

They want the physical environment of care to be one that puts them at ease.

"I woke up in ICU and it was so demoralizing. . . . I look out and you don't see anything in that room make you feel alive. You couldn't see any sky. The windows they did have were up against a brick wall."

And they want care that responds to them as a whole person, addressing not only their physical ailments, but also their psychological, emotional, spiritual, and social needs.

Staff in focus groups express that the care patients describe as ideal is, not coincidentally, the kind of care they want to deliver. They want systems that support them in providing this kind of personalized, humanized care so that they don't have to "break the rules" in order to do so.

There are growing increases in lawsuits against institutions and health professionals. Health institutions are accountable for "repairing the damage caused to consumers by deficiencies to provide the services as well as insufficient or inadequate information about their use and risks." The patient-centered assistance ensures the information and participation of patients in their treatment, helping to safeguard the institution from legal action.

—**José Henrique Germann Ferreira, MD, CEO, management consultancy, Hospital Israelita Albert Einstein, and Dr. Claudio Luiz Lottenberg, president, Sociedade Beneficiente Israelita Brasileira Albert Einstein**

PATIENT-CENTERED CARE FIELD WORK

Armed with this knowledge of how patients and caregivers define optimal care, a growing number of health care organizations are partnering with patient and family advisors to rework standard processes of care, test out innovative approaches for maximizing patient choice, autonomy, and shared decision making, and reconsider how business as usual can be reorganized to put patients first. These health care organizations, many of whom are members of the Planetree Membership Network (www. planetree.org), now with offices in the Netherlands (www.planetree.nl/), Quebec (www.reseauplanetree.org/), Brazil, Denmark, and the United States, are living laboratories where the principles of patient-centered care come alive.

This book would not exist were it not for the efforts of these living laboratories for patient-centered care, which include acute care hospitals, behavioral health settings, rehabilitation facilities, long-term care communities, home care providers, specialty hospitals, primary and ambulatory care centers, and large integrated medical systems. Together, these health care organizations are demonstrating that patient-centered care is not only an admirable aspiration, but is, in fact, a practical strategy for success in this increasingly challenged and competitive industry.

Efforts to scientifically study and measure the impact of patient-centered care implementation on a number of outcomes are promising, but they remain largely nascent. Though this work is extremely valuable and will be essential for more widespread adoption, ultimately the case for patient-centered care is not going to be made in a research institution, a laboratory, or in academia. The case for why patient-centered care is important and what it takes to successfully execute and maintain such a culture is derived from work being done in the field—in hospitals, in long-term care communities, in clinics, by practitioners, by patient and family advisers, and by site-based person-centered care task forces.

ABOUT THIS FIELD GUIDE

In this spirit, this third installment of Putting Patients First is organized as a *field guide*. In the form of illustrative case studies, patient stories, reflections on lessons learned, opportunities, and persistent challenges, this field guide encapsulates the collective wisdom of leading thinkers and practitioners of patient-centered care from around the world. You will not find a detailed history of the patient-centered care movement in these pages or the origins of the Planetree model, nor will we include a comprehensive literature review on the topic. These were covered at length in the previous two installments. The book starts with an examination of patient-centered care as a fundamental strategy for achieving high-quality, high-value care. This is followed by Part Two, in which we will transition from establishing why patient-centered care is important to the practical guidance you need to respond, on both a personal and organizational level, to the patient needs outlined earlier—for compassion, for patient-centered communication, for access to information, for family involvement, and for an environment of care that supports healing. In Part Three, contributors will impart field-tested strategies for initiating comprehensive organizational change that will last, including strategies for involving key constituent groups in the effort. Throughout the book, From Page to Practice exercises will prompt you to apply what you have learned to your own field work, and personal stories will connect you to why patient-centered care really matters.

Whether you are reading this book because you have a personal conviction that patient-centered care is the right thing to do, or you are doing so because changes to the health care landscape mean that *not* being patient-centered care is no longer an option, the questions that loom are the same: *What does it take to implement patient-centered care? How do you do it? How do you make it last?* These are precisely the questions this field guide strives to answer.

That said, this book does not purport to have all the answers for how to successfully implement patient-centered care. For as many commonalities as there are about the patient experience and the challenges facing health care organizations around the world, there are, undeniably, significant differences. The specifics of what patient-centered care looks like in practice in each unique organization are driven by the distinct needs, preferences, and experiences of the organization's key constituents—its patients, staff, leadership, community groups, regulators, payers, and competitors. No one book—not even a complete library of references—can take the place of an exchange of ideas and experiences with these groups. What we do hope, however, is that this book will support you in converting that exchange of ideas into concrete action and lasting change. Indeed, though patient-centered care is irrefutably a hot topic in health care around the globe, it is most certainly not a passing fad. We hope that this book serves as a useful companion to you on your patient-centered care journey, and is a source of ideas, inspiration, and activation for many years to come.

REFERENCES

Adams, Stephen. "NHS Patients Experience 'Contempt and Cruelty,' Says Jeremy Hunt." *Telegraph*, Nov. 28, 2012. Accessed Jan. 24, 2013, at www.telegraph.co.uk/health/healthnews/9709295/NHS-patients-experience-contempt-and-cruelty-says-Jeremy-Hunt.html

Institute of Medicine. *Crossing the Quality Chasm: A New Health System for the 21st Century*. Washington, DC: National Academy Press, 2001.

Nightingale, F. *Notes on Nursing*. New York: D. Appleton and Company, 1860.

Peabody, F. W. "The Care of the Patient." *Journal of the American Medical Association*, 1927, *88*(12), 887–882.

Schoen, C., Osborn, R., Squires, D., Doty, M., and others. "New 2011 Survey of Patients with Complex Care Needs in Eleven Countries Finds That Care Is Often Poorly Coordinated." *Health Affairs*, 2011, *30*(12), 2437–2448.

Patient-Centered Care as a Fundamental Strategy for Achieving High-Quality, High-Value Care

1

The Patient-Centered Care Value Equation

Patrick A. Charmel, Susan Stone, and Dan Otero

I retired from nursing recently, and moved to a new community, but really wanted to stay connected to my life's work in some meaningful way. I decided to volunteer at the local hospital, and was trained to be a "Care Partner" for patients who don't have family in the area to help them following a hospitalization. The hospital connected me with Shirley, a spirited, colorful, and determined sixty-eight-year-old woman who had overcome many adversities in her life. Shirley had been admitted to the hospital nine times in a ten-month period, with two of the readmissions occurring within less than a month of her previous discharge date. Her primary diagnosis was chronic obstructive pulmonary disease (COPD). She had been admitted numerous times for pneumonia, and had been prescribed a number of medications, steroids, and inhalers to control her COPD symptoms.

During one of these admissions, a Patient Activation Measure tool designed to assess patients' ability to manage their own care by examining their knowledge, skills, confidence, and readiness for change, determined that Shirley truly did not believe she had control of or confidence in managing her own medical care. Though she had previously refused all postdischarge community-based intervention offerings (including home care, hospice, and assisted living placement), the findings from this assessment made it clear that Shirley would benefit from additional support to help her understand her role in managing her health, and from coaching to do so. That was my role as her Care Partner. I visited Shirley at her home weekly and we spoke on the phone in between visits. I would ask her if she had taken her daily medications and would often find that she had forgotten her inhaler or anti-anxiety medication. Knowing of Shirley's history of anxiety, I was able to connect her to a weekly stress management clinic at the Senior Center. Following her first group session, Shirley reported to me with such relief that she went home and slept for twelve hours straight. She couldn't believe how effective just that one session was for reducing her anxiety. Over time, our relationship continued to develop, and she grew to trust me. Eventually, with supports through the hospital, I was able to convince Shirley to work with the Hospice team after her final hospital admission. Shirley did die, but she did so in her own home and on her own terms. She spent her final days surrounded by the things and people she loved, not in and out of the hospital.

—Monica

For many leaders of health care organizations around the world, the question is not whether patient-centered care is the *right* thing to do. You need only consider what you would want should you find yourself or a loved one in need of medical care to conclude that the answer to that question is an unequivocal yes. However, this decision is less clear as leaders contemplate the financial impact of adopting a patient-centered approach to care.

Stories like Shirley's, though, suggest that patient-centered care may indeed be among the most powerful levers for achieving the high-quality, high-value care that is the aim of health reform efforts worldwide. Through systems designed to assess Shirley's ability to manage her condition and interventions to engage her as a more effective steward of her own care, Shirley's last weeks and months were spent on her own terms, not being moved in and out of the hospital. From both a quality and value perspective, this was the best possible outcome—for Shirley and the hospital, alike.

At a time when global health care reform efforts are challenging providers to reduce costs while improving quality, all sensible health care leaders must consider the merits of patient-centered care both from a principled perspective and an economic one. In this chapter, through a series of field examples, we will demonstrate that patient-centered care need not come at the expense of sound fiscal management; in fact, patient-centered care can be the foundation of a successful business strategy.

FIELD EXAMPLE: **SHARP MEMORIAL HOSPITAL, SAN DIEGO, CALIFORNIA, USA**

In 2009, Sharp Memorial Hospital, a 675-bed metropolitan community hospital, had been working diligently for a number of years to improve the health care experience it provides to its patients. Since 2001 Sharp HealthCare had been on a journey to transform its organizational culture and to be the best place to work, practice, and receive care as measured by employee, physician, and patient satisfaction. In fact, Sharp Memorial Hospital had made many improvements in quality outcomes, employee satisfaction, and physician satisfaction with above-average performance

(Continued)

for all three. Patient satisfaction however, continued to lag below the 50th percentile as measured in the Press Ganey, Inc. Large Hospital Database.

Key among the strategies to improve the patient experience was using proven business exemplars such as Baldrige and the Magnet Recognition Program as roadmaps for success. In 2007, Sharp Memorial Hospital, along with the entire Sharp HealthCare organization, was recognized as a Baldrige National Quality Award–winning organization by the President of the United States. In 2008, the Magnet Recognition Program recognized Sharp Memorial Hospital as a center of nursing excellence. In 2009, Sharp Memorial Hospital added the Planetree Patient-Centered Hospital Designation criteria as an additional exemplar to guide improvement in the patient experience.

While preparing to open the new Stephen Birch Healthcare Center at Sharp Memorial Hospital, the executive team convened a group of internal stakeholders to imagine an organization that is truly responsive to the needs of employees, physicians, patients, and families. This group included team members from all levels and disciplines within the organization. They spent an entire week dreaming, imagining, and crafting a declaration creating a clear future state for all patients. The team envisioned the future where all team members would be masters in the art of caring, dedicated to creating memorable moments for every patient and becoming beacons of hope for the health care community through the demonstration of a truly transformational health care experience.

A hospital-wide collaborative patient and family-centered council conducted a self-assessment and gap analysis to determine areas of strength along with identifying the opportunities for improvement using the Patient-Centered Care Improvement Guide Self-Assessment Tool (www.patient-centeredcare.org). The gap analysis identified five priority focus areas. The Planetree organization conducted multiple focus groups with over three hundred individuals including patients, family members, staff, physicians, team members, and executives. The findings of these focus groups confirmed that much success had been made and encouraged the hospital to continue with planned program enhancements. Priority focus areas included personalized patient education, discharge preparation, increased access to health information, consistent implementation of integrative healing modalities, and parking. Table 1.1 summarizes the program enhancements implemented by the hospital-wide collaborative patient- and family-centered council.

Table 1.1 Sharp Memorial Hospital Patient- and Family-Centered Care Program Enhancements

Priority Focus Area	Patient- and Family-Centered Care Program Enhancements
Personalized patient education during hospitalization	Implementation of a television-based health information portal that converts the patient television into a computer and interactive patient education device. This program facilitates patient education and tracking as well as brings the Internet's resources and entertainment to the patient's fingertips. Implementation of the Health Information Ambassador Program to facilitate health information to the patient from the Consumer Health Library.
Discharge preparation and education	Implementation of a hospital-wide Care Partner Program to improve patient and family education and discharge preparation.
Increased access to patient health record through a shared medical record process	Creation of patient health record journal called My Health Record that allows the patient to access a summarized version of their daily medical record in order to increase patient and family participation and compliance in the care plan.

(Continued)

Table 1.1 (*Continued*)

Priority Focus Area	Patient- and Family-Centered Care Program Enhancements
Consistent implementation of integrative medicine offerings	Increased the number of integrative healing offerings in order to obtain consistent implementation throughout all units. Modalities included: • Meditation • Healing touch • Reiki • Guided imagery • Comfort hand massage • Arts for healing • Healing music • Pet therapy • Aromatherapy
Improved parking	Complimentary discharge van service for patients (one guest is permitted per patient). Purchase of a seven-passenger, wheelchair-accessible van equipped with child-safety seats.

The outcome of these patient- and family-centered program enhancements was sustained improvement in employee, physician, and patient satisfaction in addition to sustained improvement in the percentage of hospital patients assessed as receiving "perfect care" as measured by the Centers for Medicare and Medicaid Services. Sharp Memorial Hospital for the past three years outperformed 90 percent of hospitals across the United States in employee, physician, and patient satisfaction. Sharp Memorial Hospital is currently the only hospital in the world to have concurrent Planetree Patient-Centered Hospital Designation for patient-centered care excellence, Magnet designation for nursing excellence, and be part of a health care system that has received the Malcolm Baldrige

National Quality Award. In addition the following awards have demonstrated the outstanding outcomes accomplished:

- 2012 HealthExecNews World's Most Beautiful Hospital
- 2012 Becker's 100 Great Hospitals
- 2012 The Joint Commission Top Performer on Key Quality Measures
- 2011 The *Union Tribune San Diego*'s Best Hospital
- 2011 Health Grades Outstanding Patient Experience Award
- 2011 Soliant Health Top 10 America's Most Beautiful Hospitals
- 2010 Morehead Apex Award
- 2010 Soliant Health America's Most Beautiful Hospital
- 2010 Press Ganey Inpatient Top Improver Award

Figure 1.1 SMH Employee and Physician Satisfaction Percentile Rank (FY2008–FY2011)

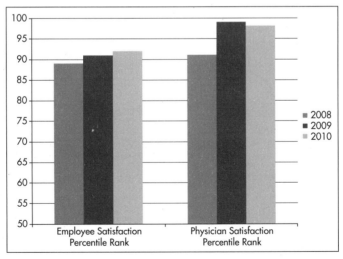

(*Continued*)

Figure 1.2 SMH Overall Patient Satisfaction Percentile Rank (FY2008–FY2011)

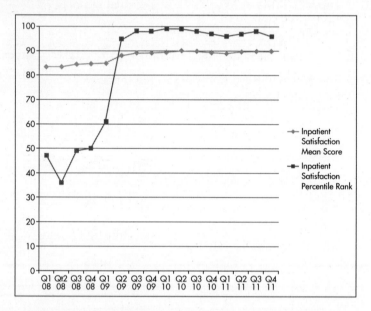

Figure 1.3 SMH Overall Percentage Perfect Care Compliance Composite (FY2008–FY2011)

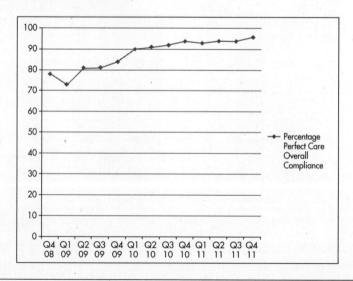

THE VALUE EQUATION

As this field example illustrates, patient-centered care and high-value health care are *not* an either-or proposition. In fact, there can be no discussion of the value equation for patient-centered care without first establishing this fundamental point: patient-centered care *is* safe, high-quality care. Health care can *not* be patient-centered if it is not grounded in clinical excellence and sound patient-safety practices.

Though the specifics of health care financing systems vary country to country, the patient-centered care value equation applies globally. It hinges on activating patients to become engaged participants in their own health care. A growing body of research demonstrates that patients who have the skills and confidence to be actively engaged in their health care:

- Are less likely to require an emergency room visit or hospital stay (Greene and Hibbard, 2012)

- Are more likely to adhere to treatment plans and manage their illness (Greene and Hibbard, 2012; Hibbard, Greene, and Overton, 2013; Remmers and others, 2009)

- Adopt healthy behavior changes (Harvey and others, 2012; Hibbard and others, 2007)

- Are associated with better health outcomes (Greene and Hibbard, 2012; Remmers and others, 2009; Skolasky, Mackenzie, Wegener, and Riley, 2011)

- Incur lower costs (Hibbard, Greene, and Overton, 2013)

In addition, numerous studies document that engaging patients drives more effective care (Beach, Keruly, and Moore, 2006; DiMatteo, 1994; DiMatteo and others, 1993; Fremont and others, 2001; Greenfield Kaplan, Ware, Yano, and Frank, 1998; Meterko, Wright, Lin, Lowy, and Cleary, 2010). When effective care is delivered, unnecessary duplication of services and readmissions are avoided, which further reduces costs.

Engaging patients as partners in their care and recognizing them as multidimensional human beings also drives patient satisfaction, which positions an organization in the marketplace as a provider of choice. In one study, researchers associated "higher perceived quality of interpersonal exchanges with physicians, greater fairness in the treatment process, and more out-of-office contact with physicians" with higher levels of patient activation (Alexander, Hearld, Mittler, and Harvey, 2012).

This relationship between a comprehensive approach to patient engagement and quality outcomes is reinforced by an examination of an elite group of hospitals that have earned recognition as Planetree Designated Patient-Centered Hospitals. These hospitals have undergone a rigorous

Figure 1.4   HCAHPS Patient Experience Survey Comparison of U.S. Designated Patient-Centered Hospitals and the National Average. *Reporting Time Period: 4/01/2011–3/31/2012*

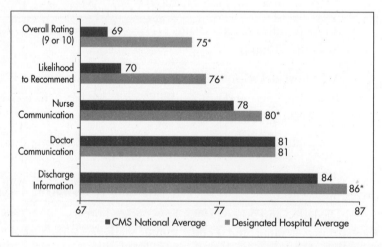

*Planetree performance is significantly better than the national average at the 95 percent confidence level (*p* < 0.05).
Note: Comparing top box scores.
Source: Hospital Compare

process to demonstrate their ability to engage patients and families, nurture staff, and deliver care in a way that meets a wide range of patient, family, and caregiver needs. Analysis of these hospitals' performance on a number of quality indicators substantiates the patient-centered care value equation. Designated Patient-Centered Hospitals in the United States consistently exceed national benchmarks for clinical quality, avoidable readmissions and patient experience.

Data further suggest that an established culture of patient-centered care accelerates improvement efforts. On the two overall measures of the patient experience included in the United States' nationally standardized Hospital Consumer Assessment of Healthcare Providers and Systems

Figure 1.5 HCAHPS Patient Experience Survey Comparison of U.S. Designated Patient-Centered Hospitals and the National Average. *Reporting Time Period: 4/01/2011–3/31/2012*

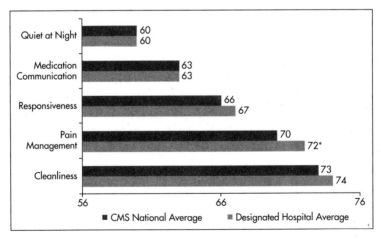

*Planetree performance is significantly better than the national average at the 95 percent confidence level (*p* < 0.05).
Note: Comparing top box scores.
Source: Hospital Compare

Figure 1.6 Percent of Patients Who Would Definitely Recommend This Hospital to Friends and Family, Rates of Improvement

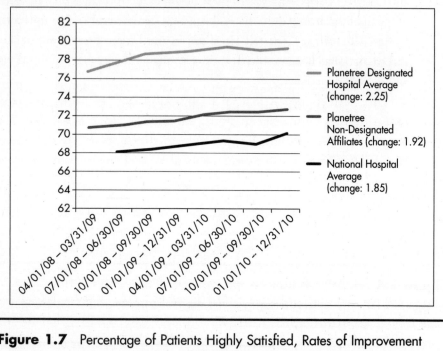

Figure 1.7 Percentage of Patients Highly Satisfied, Rates of Improvement

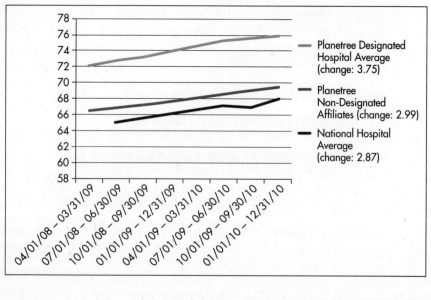

(HCAHPS) survey ("How do you rate the hospital overall?" and "Would you recommend the hospital to friends and family?"), Designated Patient-Centered Hospitals' rates of improvement exceed the national average.

Designated health care organizations in Europe and South America include some of the top-rated establishments in these regions as well. Among these is Flevoziekenhuis in The Netherlands.

FIELD EXAMPLE: **PATIENT-CENTERED QUALITY IMPROVEMENT**

Flevoziekenhuis, Almere, The Netherlands

In 2007 Flevoziekenhuis, a 268-bed acute care hospital, faced several problems, such as low performance in quality, patient satisfaction, and employee satisfaction and an unmotivated staff. This resulted in the lowest ranking of the top 100 hospitals in a national survey, a high number of patient complaints, and high employee absenteeism.

The decision to embrace the Planetree philosophy in the second half of 2007 gave the hospital a focus on improving quality from a patient and employee perspective. Measuring performance by using several methods for different purposes helped to point out the issues and problems that had to be tackled. A survey instrument was installed to continuously monitor the patient satisfaction concerning specific departments and specialists. A training program was developed for the staff after a patient survey on friendliness and hospitality in the hospital identified opportunities for improvement. Furthermore, a range of methods was offered to managers in order to improve performance, varying from focus groups to interviews in the waiting rooms. Nursing departments and outpatient clinics adopted measurement instruments based on their specific needs for information or feedback. Small groups of patients were asked for "mirror" conversations, where a large group of caregivers, doctors, and other staff experienced patients sharing their personal stories among each other, uninterrupted by staff.

(Continued)

In addition to the growing awareness of the patient experience, hospital staff focused on the importance of quality and safety standards. This led to identifying safety hazards and achieving a better registration process. Being open to identifying shortcomings facilitated overall improvement, which was quantified through yearly Planetree performance evaluations, and growing appreciation expressed by Public Health inspectors. In 2010, the hospital was ranked number one in the 100 Best Hospitals in the Country list by the national publication *Het Algemeen Dablad*. Despite the explosive growth to double its size within seven years, accompanied by a new building to accommodate the growth, the hospital managed to achieve tremendous performance improvement. Patient satisfaction increased from 6.5 in 2006 to 8.4 (on a scale of one to ten) in 2001, exceeding the national average in 2011 of 7.5. Despite the turmoil of a dynamically expanding organization, also on a scale from one to ten, employee satisfaction went from 6.2 in 2008 to 7.0 in 2010, while the percentage of employees rating themselves as "very involved" increased from 54 percent in 2008 to 73 percent in 2010. By introducing a new system of engaging doctors, nurses, and other staff in handling their patients' complaints, the number of complaints dropped from 808 in 2008 to 600 in 2010, with a further decrease of more than 20 percent in 2012. A patient survey in 2010 on the results of Planetree training showed that the hospital staff was perceived to be more friendly and hospitable than two years earlier. The year 2010 was an overall successful year. Besides the patient and staff appreciation of the Planetree implementation, Flevoziekenhuis became the first Planetree Designated Patient-Centered Hospital in Europe.

HEALTH CARE CONSUMERS ARE CHALLENGING US TO DO BETTER

As this field example attests, even countries with near-universal health care coverage are not immune to the forces of health care consumerism. Regardless of the percentage of the cost of care being paid out-of-pocket, patients recognize that decisions they make about their health care are among the most consequential they will make in their lifetimes. Accordingly, consumers are demanding more information, more choice, and greater opportunities for personal involvement in care planning and decision making.

Today's consumers are not only more informed, they are also more vocal about the quality of care they receive and their expectations of their health care delivery system. Not too long ago, a highly motivated person might write a letter of complaint—or maybe even of a letter of praise—to the CEO of a health care organization. Today, the Internet, blogs, and social media sites are forums where patients can publicly tell their stories about recent health care episodes, relating what went well and what was disappointing to them.

In addition, in many countries recent national elections have become, in essence, referendums on the state of the health care delivery system. This has driven a growing number of elected officials to examine ways to improve service quality and clinical excellence.

Elevating the Importance of the Patient Experience

The use of survey instruments to gauge patient satisfaction or the patient experience is further amplifying the voice of consumers. Such tools are gradually becoming more commonplace worldwide, and there is a growing trend for quality and patient satisfaction data to be made public, helping to inform consumers about their providers.

In the United States, the federal government—the nation's largest purchaser of health care services, through the Medicare and Medicaid programs—has mandated that hospitals report performance on a number of quality indicators, including performance on the HCAHPS survey. Until recently, hospitals that chose not to report received a substantial financial penalty. However, beginning in 2013, the reimbursement model shifted from "pay for reporting" to a "pay for performance" approach under the Medicare Value Based Purchasing (VBP) program. With the advent of value-based purchasing, how patients rate their experience of care has a very tangible impact on U.S. hospital reimbursement.

Again, hospitals with a well-established and comprehensive culture of patient-centered care are prepared to do well in a VBP environment. A preliminary analysis of the performance of the Planetree Designated Patient-Centered Hospitals on the seventeen clinical process of care measures and eight patient experience measures that comprise a hospital's value-based purchasing score forecasts that these hospitals, as a group, are poised to receive a substantial reimbursement premium. Through the VBP program, eligible hospitals will have 1 percent of their Medicare reimbursement withheld. Hospitals performing at the average will receive the entire withheld amount back. Those performing below average will only have a portion of the withheld amount returned, while above average performers will receive a greater amount than what was originally withheld. Initial indications are that Designated Patient-Centered Hospitals will receive 127 percent of the reimbursement amount held under the Value-Based Purchasing Program, indicating exceptional performance. The 27 percent premium for designated hospitals in aggregate equates to three quarters of a million dollars, which will grow as a greater portion of hospital reimbursement is tied to performance over time.

Clearly, patient-centered care can no longer be considered "value-added." It is now an obligatory component of health care organizations' strategies for financial viability. Paying health care providers based on objective measures of relative performance including the outcomes of care may manifest itself differently from country to country depending on the structure of the health care delivery system and the payment model employed, but the shift to pay for performance will no doubt occur. It is not far-fetched to suggest that, in the not too distant future, other national governments, insurance companies, and ministries of health will begin building patient experience and care effectiveness measures into their programs and reimbursement systems.

This is good news for patients. Around the world, health care leaders are mobilizing to figure out how to better respond to patient needs and preferences. In the United States, where value-based purchasing has considerably elevated the importance of patient-centered care, health care executives now identify improving the patient experience as one of their top priorities (Zeis, 2012).

Expanding Patient Choice: Medical Tourism

The growth of the medical tourism industry, wherein patients cross international borders with the express intent of obtaining more affordable or more accessible medical treatment, is further testament to how health care consumerism is altering the global health care landscape. Estimates vary considerably as to the size of the medical tourism marketplace. One group projected that the worldwide revenue generated by medical tourism would reach $100 billion by 2012 (Pizzi, 2009); another estimates the amount to be closer to $15 billion (Patients Beyond Borders, 2012). What is conclusive is that the number of patients pursuing international health care options is growing. Patients Beyond Borders (2012) estimates the annual rate of growth to be 25–35%. The rate of growth is likely to increase with the ratification of the European Union Directive on Cross Border Healthcare, which expands access to medical treatment for EU citizens in other EU nations, provided the treatment is covered in their own national health care system.

Patient-Centered Care as a Market Differentiation Strategy

Whether a health care organization sets its sights on maximizing its local market share or attracting medical tourists, many health centers today are striving to distinguish themselves from competitors. Implementation of patient-centered care can be a potent differentiator. A reputation for providing patient-centered care lends itself nicely to compelling marketing and branding efforts and word-of-mouth referrals. Even more important, the most conspicuous manifestations of patient-centered care in practice leave lasting impressions on patients and family members (for example, signage promoting shared medical records, change-of-shift caregiver to caregiver reporting at the bedside, elimination of visiting hours, elimination of overhead pages, and removal of physical barriers between patients and caregivers). These practices create the foundation for high-value care that is the ultimate focus of global health care reform efforts.

IMPROVING EFFICIENCY AND FREEING UP TIME TO CARE

This emphasis on value has resulted in many health care organizations scrutinizing operating costs and resource allocation in order to eliminate waste and inefficiencies. Process improvement to make organizations "leaner" has proven to be immensely effective in other industries and sectors, resulting in greater efficiency and productivity and increased return on investment. To be sure, the health care industry is hardly immune to waste. A focus on value, undeniably, requires health care leaders to seek out opportunities for reductions in costs and elimination of redundancy and inefficiency. However, unlike a manufacturer whose commodity is widgets, our commodities in health care are the restoration of health and well-being of individuals at among the most vulnerable times in their lives. The questions of cost, productivity, and efficiency must be considered in the context of the human experience. Such is the focus of the Patient-Centered (PC) Lean process improvement approach.

Patient-Centered Lean combines established lean methodologies with the principles of patient-centered care to realize the patient-centered care value equation. The methodologies focus in on ways to improve the patient experience, optimize work flows, reduce rework and defects, and increase financial returns, all while activating patients as partners in their care and heightening staff engagement and morale.

PC Lean initiatives examine several core performance drivers to realize superior and consistent returns:

- *Staff and patient driven:* Employees and patients contribute to Lean events, results produced, and time invested in the process

- *Leadership supported:* Executive leadership leads the way by ensuring resource allocation, removing barriers to success, and celebrating accomplishments with the Patient-Centered Lean team

- *Value stream selection and results tracking:* The alignment of strategic planning, patient-centered care methodology, and critical organizational goals; project scope and boundaries; matching the right resources and tools; and accurately measuring improvements

- *Ability to replicate improvements:* Ways that solutions and standard work can be applied across multiple departments throughout the organization

- *Sustainability and performance management:* Ensuring that solutions are sustained over time through daily management of standard work

---

FIELD EXAMPLE: **PATIENT-CENTERED LEAN IN PRACTICE**

Griffin Hospital, Derby, Connecticut, USA

Griffin Hospital is a 160-bed acute care hospital located in the highly competitive health care market of the northeastern United States. Although there are a number of larger and better-known health care institutions in close proximity, Griffin has gained a reputation as a hospital of choice, known for engaging patients and families through access to information, shared decision making, and encouraging their active involvement in organizational planning and improvement efforts. At the same time, the hospital has emerged as an employer of choice for its efforts to care for and support staff so that they can best care for and support patients.

The Griffin Hospital story illustrates how a focused effort to reorganize care delivery around the experience of patients can improve clinical, operational, and financial outcomes. Once a struggling hospital with a deteriorating physical plant, a reputation as a hospital to be avoided, and an uncertain future, today the hospital is a patient-centered care success story.

Systemic culture change began more than twenty years ago with a concerted effort to listen to employees and patients and respond in

(*Continued*)

meaningful ways to their needs and preferences. Retreats reconnected all employees to why being a health care professional mattered to them. These mandatory overnight, off-site retreats also created a foundation where every employee, clinical and nonclinical alike, views themselves as caregivers with the ability and responsibility to deliver an exceptional patient experience. Focus groups, patient surveys, and community image surveys became vital tools for charting the course for how care would be delivered moving forward.

A shared medical record policy, health resource centers, a care partner program, patient pathways, and collaborative care conferences were introduced to ensure that patients and their families have access to the information they need to be partners in decisions about their care, treatment, and well-being. Featuring residential kitchens, healing artwork, family lounges, decentralized nurses' stations right outside of patient rooms, consumer health libraries on every unit, abundant natural light, and access to nature, the physical environment also reflects patient-centered care principles.

By putting patients first, the hospital dramatically changed its trajectory from a struggling institution to one that is thriving and has earned a reputation for excellence on multiple fronts. In the most recently completed survey, of the eight hospitals in its region, Griffin was named the hospital of choice by community residents and identified as the most improved hospital by a three-to-one margin. Patient satisfaction has averaged 96 percent for the past five years. In 2011, Griffin Hospital was named one of the top performing hospitals in the United States on key quality measures by The Joint Commission, the leading accreditor of health care organizations in the United States. The hospital is in the top 5 percent of all U.S. hospitals recognized for consistent, comprehensive quality outcomes across several medical specialties. It is also the only hospital to have been named on *Fortune* magazine's "100 Best Companies to Work For" list for ten consecutive years.

Fundamental to Griffin Hospital's success has been its commitment to continuous improvement. Given narrowing operating margins and health care reform that has transformed financial incentives, perhaps never in the hospital's history has this ability to innovate, evolve, and improve been more important.

While the Griffin team endeavors to transform how it operates, what will remain unchanged is its central focus on the patient. Through deployment of the Patient-Centered Lean process, the hospital has initiated numerous projects in several departments which are projected to save more than $400,000 annually by increasing efficiencies and capturing additional revenue—all while simultaneously enhancing the patient experience.

The Griffin Hospital team initiated its strategic deployment of PC Lean with one overarching goal in mind: to get the caregiver back at the bedside where value is added. This strategic goal started the deployment that led Inpatient, Surgical, Emergency, Laboratory, Case Management, and Human Resources to integrate their improvement efforts. These efforts led to improved staff engagement, quality, safety, access and timely delivery of care, and financial returns as well as reduced operating costs and increased capacity. Just a small sampling of the changes implemented include:

- The nursing care delivery model was redesigned to better promote accountability and team work, with the ultimate intent of enhancing responsiveness to patients' needs. With the establishment of a consistent shift start time, all oncoming staff (including the charge nurse, RNs, multiskilled technicians, and the unit clerk) now begin their shift together with a brief team meeting during which the unit's patients are reviewed and team members' work assignments are established. In this new model of care, each team member's daily responsibilities are conditional on what is occurring on the unit that day versus rigid job descriptions that narrowly define certain tasks for nurses and others for techs. Processes were also implemented to ensure that, even with multiple shifts (four-hour, eight-hour, and twelve-hour), the patient's vital role on the care team is not overlooked. It was established that every eight hours, the patient be a part of the team meeting. In addition, in an

(Continued)

initiative driven by the multiskilled technicians, a formalized protocol was devised for ensuring that patients' call lights are directed to the appropriate level of care based on the type of request, and that the lights are responded to in a timely manner.

- The preoperative interview and admission testing procedures for same-day surgery patients was restructured. In the new process, pre-op patient interviews are conducted over the phone versus in person, saving the patient an extra trip to the hospital. In addition, pre-op testing is now provided on a walk-in basis, whereas previously such tests needed to be scheduled. This provides patients with greater flexibility. Additional improvements were instituted to minimize the burden on patients requiring more extensive pre-op work that cannot be done on a walk-in basis. By having the anesthesiology team reserve a consistent block of time when they are available, schedulers are able to be more efficient in coordinating patients' care and managing staff's time.

- A new discharge process introduced in the Emergency Department established a standardized core set of responsibilities in the discharge process. By having the physician print off the discharge instructions and physically drop them in a bin at the nurses' station, nurses are visually cued, in a time-efficient way, when their patient has been cleared for discharge so that they can print off the discharge instructions, reducing the time between the physician entering a discharge order and the actual discharge of the patient.

- The daily workflow of staff in the Case Management Department was made more efficient by streamlining the department's customary morning briefing. What was previously a meeting that took anywhere from forty-five to sixty minutes was pared down to just fifteen minutes by eliminating interruptions (phones are answered by the clerk) and standardizing the information to be exchanged. By reducing the time of this important administrative process, case managers are freed up to spend more time meeting with patients and family members earlier on in their work day. This significant reduction in the time of the daily briefing has been realized even with the inclusion of a reflection at the start of every briefing to center staff and start the day on an uplifting and supportive note.

- Space in the surgical preoperative area being used as a storage area was repurposed and redesigned to use as patient care space. Recognizing the healing benefits of natural light, the space was reconfigured to bring more outside light into the area.

Through implementation of these changes, the hospital is poised to:

- Save nearly seven hundred nurse hours per year
- Recoup useable space valued at $98,000 annually
- Increase capacity
- Improve employee satisfaction

Improvement in patient and family satisfaction is also being driven through these process improvements. The patient experience has been enhanced through:

- Maximizing nurses' time at the bedside
- Minimizing discharge delays
- Decreasing the wait time for same-day surgery patient interviews
- Reducing Emergency Department wait times from patient arrival to when the patient is seen by a physician
- Reducing admission times from the Emergency Department to the inpatient unit
- Incorporating into the standardized Emergency Department discharge process a bedside discharge brief which involves the patient so that they have a better understanding of the discharge process and their discharge instructions

With an eye on sustaining these improvements, the hospital has developed visual tools and reports to help all team members gauge performance and maintain these early gains.

CONCLUSION

Limited resources and mounting financial pressures challenge all of today's health care leaders. As demonstrated in this chapter, engaging patients and families through a person-centered approach to care represents an unparalleled opportunity to achieve the high-quality, high-value care we all strive to deliver.

REFERENCES

Alexander, J. A., Hearld, L. R., Mittler, J. N., and Harvey, J. "Patient-Physician Role Relationships and Patient Activation Among Individuals with Chronic Illness." *Health Services Research*, 2012 June, *47*(3 Pt. 1), 1201–1223.

Beach, M. C., Keruly, J., and Moore, R. D. "Is the Quality of the Patient-Provider Relationship Associated with Better Adherence and Health Outcomes for Patients with HIV?" *Journal of General Internal Medicine*, 2006, *21*(6), 661–665.

DiMatteo, M. R. "Enhancing Patient Experience to Medical Recommendations." *Journal of the American Medical Association*, 1994, *271*(1), 79, 83.

DiMatteo, M. R., Sherbourne, C. D., Hays, R. D., Ordway, L., and others. "Physicians' Characteristics Influence Patients' Adherence to Medical Treatment: Results from the Medical Outcomes Study." *Health Psychology*, 1993, *12*(2), 93–102.

Fremont, A. M., Cleary, P. D., Hargraves, J. L., Rowe, R. M., and others. "Patient-Centered Processes of Care and Long-Term Outcomes of Acute Myocardial Infarction." *Journal of General Internal Medicine*, 2001, *16*(12), 800–808.

Greene, J., and Hibbard, J. H. "Why Does Patient Activation Matter? An Examination of the Relationships Between Patient Activation and Health-Related Outcomes." *Journal of General Internal Medicine*, 2012, *27*(5), 520–526.

Greenfield, S., Kaplan, H. S., Ware, J. E. Jr., Yano, E. M., and others. "Patients' Participation in Medical Care: Effects on Blood Sugar Control and Quality of Life in Diabetes." *Journal of General Internal Medicine*, 1998, *3*(5) 448–457.

Harvey, L., Fowles, J. B., Xi, M., and Terry, P. "When Activation Changes, What Else Changes? The Relationship Between Change in Patient Activation Measure (PAM) and Employees' Health Status and Health Behaviors." *Patient Education and Counseling*, 2012, *88*(2), 338–343.

Hibbard, J. H., Greene, J., and Overton, V. "Patients with Lower Activation Associated with Higher Costs: Delivery Systems Should Know Their Patients' 'Scores.'" *Health Affairs*, 2013, *32*(2), 216–222.

Hibbard, J. H., Mahoney, E. R., Stock, R., and Tusler, M. "Do Increases in Patient Activation Result in Improved Self-Management Behaviors?" *Health Services Research*, 2007, *42*(4), 1443–1463.

Meterko, M., Wright, S., Lin, H., Lowy, E., and Cleary, P. D. "Mortality Among Patients with Acute Myocardial Infarction: the Influences of Patient-Centered Care and Evidence-Based Medicine." *Health Services Research*, 2010, *45*(5), 1188–1204.

Patients Beyond Borders. "Medical Tourism Statistics and Facts." Accessed Oct. 1, 2012, at www.patientsbeyondborders.com/medical-tourism-statistics-facts

Pizzi, R. "Global Medical Tourism Revenue to Hit $100B by 2012." *Healthcare Finance News*, June 29, 2009. Accessed April 2013 at www.healthcarefinancenews.com/news/global-medical-tourism-revenue-hit-100b-2012

Remmers, C., Hibbard, J., Mosen, D. M., Wagenfield, M., and others. "Is Patient Activation Associated with Future Health Outcomes and Healthcare Utilization Among Patients with Diabetes?" *Journal of Ambulatory Care Management*, 2009, *32*(4), 1–8.

Skolasky, R. L., Mackenzie, E. J., Wegener, S. T., and Riley, L. H. "Patient Activation and Functional Recovery in Persons Undergoing Spine Surgery." *Orthopedics*, 2011, *34*(11), 888.

Zeis, M. "Patient Experience and HCAHPS: Little Consensus on a Top Priority." Accessed August 2012 at www.healthleadersmedia.com/intelligence/detail.cfm?content_id=282893&year=2012

2

Defining and Measuring Patient-Centered Quality

Sara Guastello, Marcel Snijders, Róisín Boland, and Paula Wilson

On my first day of chemotherapy, I had both new medicine and so many different emotions coursing through my body. I was scared, nervous, sad, overwhelmed, and anxious. But I was also hopeful that this was the beginning of my healing process. To literally put my life in the hands of my doctors and nurses was such an unfamiliar state of being for me. I'm an independent person, and I've never before had any serious health issues. When I was diagnosed, I felt that I was no longer in the driver's seat of my own life. Never before had I felt so out of control of my own future. Reflecting back on that first day of chemotherapy, though, one nurse's actions stand out in my mind. She took the time to sit with me before my treatment and answer all my questions, and she did so without making me feel spoken down to or patronized. If I didn't understand her answer, I asked her to clarify, and she did, never making me feel that I was being a nuisance by wanting information. In fact, when I told her I was out of questions, she said, "Are you sure? I have the time to answer whatever questions you have." The nurse not only answered all of my questions about the chemo meds, she also printed out all the information about the medications.

Three months later, I was invited to participate in a focus group at the hospital to share my story and ideas for improving the care experience. During the focus group, I recalled this interaction with the nurse and told the group how impressed I was that she took the time to do that. That is so important because you want a certain level of control. When they do bring you information to read about your treatment it really adds to your level of confidence.

Beyond the sharing of information, what meant the most to me was the compassion I felt from the nurse. When she saw that I was becoming emotional at the thought of the road ahead, she gently touched my arm and offered words of reassurance. That gentle gesture spoke volumes. That touch made me feel that I was in good hands, and that for this nurse, I was not just a patient, but a person.
—Abel

DEFINING PATIENT-CENTERED CARE

Though most patients would be hard-pressed to recite a formal definition of patient-centered care, as Abel's story attests, when patient-centeredness is experienced, it leaves a powerful and positive impression. Nonetheless, as adoption of patient-centered care spreads worldwide—sought out by patients and health care professionals alike—it becomes increasingly important to define what one can expect from a patient-centered provider. Otherwise, the term risks becoming a meaningless descriptor for product advertisements and mission statements that fails to make a real difference for patients and those who care for them.

Numerous definitions for patient-centered care exist. At their core, all of these definitions emphasize partnership, patient responsibility and participation in their care:

Health care that establishes a partnership among practitioners, patients and their families (when appropriate) to ensure that decisions respect patients' wants, needs, and preferences and that patients have the education and support they require to make decisions and participate in their own care. (Institute of Medicine, 2001)

The essence of patient-centred healthcare is that the healthcare system is designed and delivered to address the healthcare needs and preferences of patients so that healthcare is appropriate and cost-effective. By promoting greater patient responsibility and optimal usage, patient-centred healthcare leads to improved health outcomes, quality of life and optimal value for healthcare investment. (International Alliance of Patients' Organizations, 2006)

Care organized around the patient . . . a model in which providers partner with patients and families to identify and satisfy the full range of patient needs and preferences. (Planetree and Picker Institute, 2008)

THE TIE THAT BINDS QUALITY, SAFETY, AND THE PATIENT EXPERIENCE

These definitions firmly shift patient-centered care beyond the realm of amenities and hospitality to a fundamental dimension of quality. By emphasizing effective partnerships and communication and honoring patients' individuality and humanity, an organizational culture of person-centered care not only measurably enhances the patient experience, but also creates a strong basis for overall clinical quality and patient safety. This relationship between patient experience and quality is apparent in the findings of a 2011 study which found that hospitals' performance on the Hospital Consumer Assessment of Healthcare Providers and

Systems (HCAHPS) patient experience survey was more predictive of readmission rates "than the objective clinical performance measures often used to assess the quality of hospital care" (Boulding and others, 2011).

Building on this relationship, a growing number of health care accrediting bodies (long seen as the preeminent arbiters of health care quality and safety) are incorporating patient-centered care into their standards and accreditation processes. According to the International Society for Quality in Health Care (ISQua), which operates the only global external evaluation program specific to health care that "accredits the accreditors," accreditation/external evaluation organizations worldwide are increasingly becoming more patient-centered with a particular focus in the collection and use of patient feedback for the purpose of quality improvement to ensure that care and service delivery meets their needs.

Among these accrediting bodies that have embedded patient-centered care into their standards is Joint Commission International (JCI), the international arm of The Joint Commission and accreditor/certifier of more than 540 health care organizations in over fifty countries (as of 2012). Reflecting this growing recognition that patient-centered care cannot be separated out from quality and safety, JCI has incorporated standards focusing the hospital staff on the importance of building a trusting relationship with the patient and the importance of embracing the cultural, psychosocial, and spiritual values of patients and their families. Though on the surface, this may appear to be outside of the realm of quality, the inclusion of these standards underscores that establishing rapport and getting to know patients beyond their diagnosis and treatment plans is not only the heart of patient-centered care, but also the foundation for quality.

The connection between patient-centered care and quality is reinforced through additional standards that make clear that the patient and family should be informed about what the plan of care is and what outcomes can be expected from the care. No care should be rendered without the informed consent of the patient. This also means that the patient and family should receive education and information about all of their choices and the risks associated with various treatment options. Throughout JCI's 320 international accreditation standards, the importance of communicating in the patient's language and being respectful of the patient's culture and beliefs is stressed, further underscoring the interconnectivity between patient-centered care and quality.

Beyond the adoption of patient-centered standards, other accrediting bodies, such as Accreditation Canada, have incorporated a distinctly patient-centered (or client-centered) focus to the entirety of the accreditation process. A distinctive feature of Accreditation Canada's Qmentum program is the scope of services assessed. Organizations are evaluated and accredited as clients or patients actually experience care. Across the different Canadian provinces and territories, the client experience spans multiple points of care, and fundamental to high-quality care delivery is the coordination and communication among various services and sectors. Accreditation Canada has adopted a system-level approach to accreditation, defining the scope as inclusive of all the health care services within the organization. This approach supports health care systems in providing the best possible care to meet the needs of clients and patients as they transition across the continuum.

With client-centered standards pertaining to both leadership and clinical teams across the organization, the Qmentum accreditation program emphasizes that client-centered care is most effective when processes are in place throughout the system to support patient and family engagement. This approach necessitates that organizations involve community members in strategic planning as they map out future directions while at the same time supporting individual clients during care in being active, informed, and engaged.

Despite the differences among health care accrediting bodies worldwide, the fundamental purpose of them all is to improve quality in health care. By adopting a more patient-centered focus to how they evaluate quality, a number of accrediting bodies are transforming patient-centered care into an essential dimension of how quality is defined.

THE BIG QUESTION

Despite the fact that patient-centered care is increasingly included as part of the safety and quality agendas of individual provider organizations, accrediting bodies, and health care systems as a whole, there is still a disconnect. An analysis of quality rankings of health care systems of industrialized nations around the world demonstrates that a high ranking for overall quality does not necessarily translate into a high ranking for patient-centeredness (Davis, Schoen, and Stremikis, 2010). Similarly, a 2010 analysis of U.S. hospitals' performance on the standardized quality of care and patient experience measures that now dictate a portion of hospitals' reimbursement found that hospitals' greatest opportunity for maximizing reimbursement was not related to improvement in traditional and technical measures of quality. The greatest opportunity for improvement was related to the patient experience (Healthcare Financial Management Association, 2010).

This begs the question: *Why do health care organizations that excel in other dimensions of quality and safety continue to struggle to deliver patient-centered care?* The answer may very well lie in the experiences of organizations that rank highly in both traditional measures of quality *and* patient-centeredness. For these organizations, patient-centered care is not a happy coincidence fueled by good intentions. It is a deliberate, focused, and strategic organizational priority guided by a concrete framework and subject to measurement to ensure steady progress and guard against complacency.

RAISING THE BAR IN PATIENT-CENTERED CARE THROUGH DESIGNATION

Such is the case for the hospitals and long-term care communities that have achieved Planetree Designation as Patient-Centered Hospitals or Resident-Centered Communities. A comprehensive program for evaluating patient-centered care, the Patient-Centered Hospital Designation

Program is the only program that formally recognizes person-centered excellence across the continuum of care.

The criteria that an organization must satisfy to be awarded designation are based on extensive focus group research with thousands of patients, family members, and health care professionals about how they define patient-centered quality. The criteria include a shared medical record policy, nonrestrictive visiting practices, opportunities for patient and family input into health center operations, healthy and flexible meal options, recognition of the role of spirituality and the arts in healing, and a physical environment that facilitates privacy, promotes open communication between patients and providers, and is accommodating of family members' involvement in their loved one's care. Recognizing that ultimately the patient experience originates with those providing care, several criteria focus on nurturing a work environment that is supportive of staff.

Focus groups with stakeholders ensure that designated hospitals, long-term care communities, and primary care centers are not only able to document their patient-centered practices, but that the effectiveness of the practices is validated by those they are intended to benefit. This focus group work is the basis of designation decisions, and more importantly, it guides applicant sites' ongoing improvement efforts.

The designation criteria represent a nonprescriptive framework for culture change, showing what patient-centered excellence looks like without dictating a one-size-fits-all formula for success. Thus, each organization striving for designation approaches its culture change journey and implements strategies that are congruent with its distinct realities, including its current financial, cultural, and environmental state.

The Relationship Between Designation and Accreditation

The Patient-Centered Hospital Designation Program differs from traditional health care quality accreditations in its scope. While there is a fair amount of overlap in general areas covered (safety, governance, disclosure, patient education, outcomes), how excellence is defined and evaluated differs. For instance, traditional accreditation standards evaluate the physical environment from the perspective of access, safety and emergency management. The Patient-Centered Hospital Designation Program offers a complementary set of criteria that focus on how the environment promotes healing and reduces stress, such as appropriate wayfinding, attention to noise levels, maximizing privacy, appropriate space for families, and access to nature. Both approaches are important, and both are focused on the patient; one does not preclude the other. In fact, in many cases as demonstrated by the example above, there is an elegant harmony between national and international accreditation standards and the designation criteria. Progress on one will propel progress toward the other, all while taking an organization to new heights of quality.

From Page to Practice: Planetree International Designation Readiness Assessment

The tool below is designed to assist organizations in determining their readiness to apply for Patient-Centered Designation as well as to identify priorities as you progress in your culture change journey. To complete the readiness assessment, rate your organization's current status on each element based on the following scale:

Fully implemented throughout the organization
- Fully integrated into the organization
- On all units
- On all shifts

Partially implemented
- On some units, but not all
- On some shifts, but not all
- Implementation is in progress, but not yet fully integrated into the organization

No activity
- No progress has been made related to the element

Table 2.1 Patient-Centered Hospital Designation Readiness Assessment

	Fully Implemented Throughout Organization	Partially Implemented	No Activity	N/A
1 The organization's commitment to patient-centered care is reflected in its mission statement.				
2 The multidisciplinary team established to oversee patient-centered care implementation includes a balance of nonsupervisory and management staff.				
3 An active Patient and Family Advisory Council is in place and provides input on current practices and new initiatives.				
4 All staff have had the opportunity to participate in experiential training (such as a retreat) to sensitize them to the patient experience.				
5 Systems are in place to regularly educate physicians about the organization's patient-centered initiatives.				
6 Job descriptions and performance evaluations include competencies related to patient-centered care.				

(Continued)

Table 2.1 (Continued)

	Fully Implemented Throughout Organization	Partially Implemented	No Activity	N/A
7 Staff at all levels, clinical and nonclinical, have the opportunity to voice their ideas and suggestions for improvement.				
8 Space away from patients and families is available for staff to decompress between patients or cases.				
9 Patients are able to review their active medical record, care plan, or equivalent and there is support available to assist them in understanding the content.				
10 Patient education materials appropriate for readers of varying literacy levels and for speakers of different native languages are readily available.				
11 Plans of care are written in language that patients and families can understand.				

12 Protocols are in place for fully disclosing unanticipated outcomes to patients (and family members, as appropriate).

13 Flexible, 24-hour patient-directed visiting hours are in place hospital-wide, including in the ICU.

14 Comfortable spaces are available for family use.

15 Patients have a choice of what to eat *and* when to eat.

16 Healthy food is available to all staff, including those who work on weekends and at night.

17 In your most recent renovation or construction project, users of the space were involved in the design process.

18 Patients have choices or control over their personal environment, including thermal comfort, visual privacy, and noises and sounds.

19 Patients have access to a variety of arts and entertainment.

20 Systems are in place to integrate patients' spiritual beliefs into their care and treatment.

(Continued)

Table 2.1 (Continued)

	Fully Implemented Throughout Organization	Partially Implemented	No Activity	N/A
21	A broad range of healing modalities, including those considered complementary to Western or traditional modalities, are offered to meet the needs of patients.			
22	The organization collaborates with local agencies on provision of direct services, educational information, or referral.			
23	Data are gathered to measure patient safety and are used to inform improvement efforts.			
24	Data are gathered to measure the patient experience and are used to inform improvement efforts.			
25	Data are gathered to measure the staff experience and are used to inform improvement efforts.			

MEASURING PATIENT-CENTEREDNESS

Evidence compiled since the launch of the Patient-Centered Hospital Designation Program in 2007 demonstrates that the designation framework not only supports sustained culture change, but also improves outcomes. Designation is associated with superior performance in clinical quality measures and patient experience measures (Frampton and Guastello, 2010). Also considered as part of the designation process are employee experience survey data, turnover rates, and performance on culture of safety surveys. Embedding measurement into the Patient-Centered Hospital Designation Program required many thoughtful and challenging questions about how to measure person-centeredness.

As patient-centered care has gained prominence as a critical dimension of health care quality, efforts to measure it have begun to flourish around the globe. In the United States, the HCAHPS survey serves as a standardized measure of the patient experience. Hospitals' performance on the survey is publicly reported, along with national benchmarks. Incorporating HCAHPS performance into the equation that determines hospitals' reimbursement further elevates the importance of the patient experience as a driver of quality, high-value care. Elsewhere in the world, patient experience surveys such as the Consumer Quality Index (CQI) in the Netherlands and the Picker Patient Satisfaction Survey in Europe are emerging as important instruments for measuring the patient experience and involving patients in assessing patient-centered quality.

The use of patient experience surveys, though, is just one approach for measuring patient-centeredness. Given the complexity of person-centered culture change, one would be best suited to take a multidimensional approach to measurement. Table 2.2 illustrates a variety of measures that could be incorporated to identify successes, gauge progress, and ascertain opportunities for improvement in the culture change journey.

It stands to reason that any approach for the measurement of person-centeredness must include patient-reported measures, such as the patient experience surveys, health confidence measures, patient-reported outcomes measures and health-related quality-of-life measures listed in Table 2.2.

Table 2.2 Measures to Assess Aspects of Patient-Centered Care

Measure Type	Examples	Considerations
Patient experience surveys	• HCAHPS, CQI, Picker Patient Satisfaction Survey • Net Promoter Score (NPS) • Conseil Québécois d'Agrément; Accreditation Canada	• Standardized questions and data collection methodologies enable benchmarking and trending an organization's performance over time. • Questions may be limited in scope, failing to capture the depth and complexity of the patient experience.
Qualitative data	• Focus groups • Patient interviews • Testimonials, letters of compliment or complaint	• Captures patients' stories, experiences, and ideas in more depth than surveys are able to do. • By connecting patient-centered care to personal stories, can become very powerful tools for inspiring caregivers and igniting change. • Cannot be trended over time or compared to benchmarks in any systematic way.
Traditional quality metrics	• Process of care indicators • Readmission rates • Infection rates • Adherence rates • Mortality rates	• Reinforce the connections between patient-centered care and quality. • Data points are generally already being captured. • Lack the patient perspective.

Quality of care transitions	• Care Transitions Measure (CTM-3; CTM-15)
	• Measures patient experiences with care coordination when leaving a hospital setting.
	• The three-item measure (CTM-3) has low response burden.
	• Used in 15 countries worldwide. A Spanish version is available.
	• As of January 1, 2013, CMS is mandating that U.S. hospitals currently participating in the HCAHPS data submission use the Expanded HCAHPS Survey which includes the CTM-3.
Empathy	• Jefferson Scale of Physician/ Medical Student/Health Professionals Empathy (JSPE) • Person-Centred Climate Questionnaire-Patient Version (PCQ-P) (Edvardsson, Koch, and Nay, 2009); Person-Centred Climate Questionnaire-Staff Version (PCQ-S) (Edvardsson, Koch, and Nay, 2010)
	• The JSPE is a psychometrically reliable instrument to measure empathy in the context of medical education and patient care.
	• The JSPE is available in 38 languages and has been used in 54 countries worldwide.
	• JSPE Scales are not designed to measure empathy of nonclinical/ancillary staff.
	• Person-Centered Climate Questionnaire designed to assess perceptions of person-centeredness of health care setting by both patients and staff.

(Continued)

Table 2.2 (Continued)

Measure Type	Examples	Considerations
Employee experience, compassion satisfaction, fatigue, burnout	• Employee experience and satisfaction surveys • Professional Quality of Life Scale fourth version (ProQOL R-IV) • National Consensus Project to define compassionate healthcare by the Schwartz Center • Self-Compassion Scale (SCS) (Neff, 2003)	• The ProQOL is recommended for screening for compassion fatigue and burnout, but not diagnosis. The tool is available in 17 languages. • The National Consensus Project is a recently funded initiative through the Arthur Vining Davis Foundation to develop definitions and measures of compassionate health care. Materials are under development at the time of this publication. • The SCS is a 26-item measure tapping self-kindness, self-judgment, common humanity, isolation, mindfulness, and over-identification. Participants respond to various items about "how I typically act toward myself in difficult times" on a 5-point scale, with higher total scores indicating greater self-compassion.
Patient-reported outcomes measures (PROMs)	• Sweden's rheumatoid arthritis registry, which collects patient-reported data on joint pain, current health status, and quality of life	• Focus on individual patients' perceptions of their own health status. • Can be incorporated into a patient's plan of care and then used to track the impact of the care plan on outcomes. • Adoption of such measures remains limited in scope at present, though efforts to expand use are promising.

Health confidence measures	• Patient Activation Measure (PAM)	• Patient-reported measure of the extent to which patients have the knowledge, skills, and confidence to manage their health (Greene and Hibbard, 2012).
Health-related quality of life	• Includes domains related to physical, mental, emotional, and social functioning; such as HRQoL, SF-36 health survey • Personal Health Inventory ("My Story") in Veteran's Health Administration • Assessment of Life Habits (LIFE-H); MHAVIE (French) • Satisfaction With Life Scale (SWLS)	• Focuses on impact health status has on quality of life. Bridges the full continuum of care and support services. • Validity and reliability tests of the SF-36 have been conducted in older populations, primary care, and community settings. Available in Spanish. • PHI is a web-based application that allows veterans and military men and women to define their health goals important for their quality of life. • The LIFE-H covers many domains of life similar to the WHO International Classification of Functioning, Disability and Health (ICF) domains. • The Satisfaction With Life Scale (SWLS) measures the individual's evaluation of satisfaction with his life in general. Life satisfaction is an important factor of subjective well-being (with positive affective appraisal and negative affective appraisal) and is more cognitively than emotionally driven.

(Continued)

Table 2.2 (Continued)

Measure Type	Examples	Considerations
Symptom/ symptom burden	• The HRQoL includes a Healthy Days Symptom Module and Activity Limitation measure available through the Centers for Disease Control (CDC). Disease-specific questionnaires are widely available.	• Symptom burden surveys can be used to understand specific disease burdens among patients with comorbidities (for example, diabetes and depression) in specialized care settings, such as receiving palliative care or children's hospitals.
Health-related behaviors	• Examples include the Department of Defense Health Related Behaviors (HRB) for active duty military personnel.	• Includes lifestyle assessments, such as alcohol, drug, and tobacco use, which can be used to identify at-risk patients and codevelop patient-centered interventions.

Not only is it fitting, but one could easily argue that *not* including patient-reported measures undermines any efforts to delivery truly patient-centered care. Nonetheless, the adoption of patient-reported quality measures remains a daunting proposition for many providers. Patients, some may argue, do not grasp the complexities or nuances of health care, and may have unrealistic expectations. A growing body of literature suggests, however, that patients are astute judges of health care quality. Numerous studies show higher scores on patient experience measures correlate with higher scores on clinical quality indicators (Glickman and others, 2010; Isaac and others, 2010).

Measurement Challenges

Sound measurement systems drive internal quality improvement efforts and enable organizations to respond to the increasing demand from the government, health insurance companies, patients, and potential employees for data to demonstrate quality in an increasingly competitive health care market. Just as measurement has the potential to drive quality, so too can it thwart improvement efforts when systems and instruments are poorly developed, frequently changed, misused, or misinterpreted.

For instance, in the Netherlands quality rankings of the country's one hundred hospitals are published annually by two newspapers and one magazine. Each publication uses slightly different calculations and criteria to compute its rankings, and the criteria have been changed from year to year. As a result, in the same year, a Dutch hospital was ranked number one in the country by one newspaper and eightieth in another. In another example, a hospital dropped in an annual ranking from number one to number fifty the following year in the same paper due to changing criteria and a lack of adequate source information. Discrepancies like these cause confusion for patients, frustrate leaders, demoralize staff, and create a scenario in which this publicly reported quality information creates more questions than it answers.

Complementing quantitative performance data with qualitative data can paint a more complete picture of the patient and staff experience in an organization. Focus groups, rounding, and mystery shopper programs are just a few ways that health care organizations are soliciting the opinions and ideas of their stakeholders. Planetree Nederland has devised a system for quantifying focus group findings. Every eighteen months, focus group participants are asked to rate their experiences at an organization with each of the components of the Planetree model (for instance, human interactions, access to information, family involvement), as well their perception of the importance of that particular component. Participants also use a 10-point scale to rate their overall satisfaction, the "human atmosphere," the "ambition" of the organization, and their willingness to recommend a family member or friend to the organization. Scores are analyzed to identify any areas of regression or where the organization may benefit from adapting work processes or policies.

CONCLUSION: A GOAL THAT CAN BE SET, MEASURED, AND ACHIEVED

Today organizations have more tools than ever before to gauge progress in their pursuit of patient-centered excellence. Supporting this aim are the development of patient experience survey instruments, patient-reported quality measures, and more accreditation and external evaluation organizations embedding patient-centered care principles into their standards and evaluation processes. In addition, a growing number of health care organizations are using the Patient-Centered Hospital Designation criteria as a blueprint *and* measure for their culture change journey. Though challenges around defining and measuring patient-centeredness persist, the efforts described in this chapter have contributed toward converting patient-centered care from a vague and elusive aim into a goal that can be set, measured, and achieved.

REFERENCES

Boulding, W., Glickman, S. W., Manary, M. P., Schulman, K. A., and others. "Relationship Between Patient Satisfaction with Inpatient Care and Hospital

Readmission Within 30 Days." *American Journal of Managed Care*, 2011, *17*(1), 41–48.

Davis, K., Schoen, C., and Stremikis, K. *Mirror, Mirror on the Wall: How the Performance of the U.S. Health Care System Compares Internationally 2010 Update*. New York: Commonwealth Fund, June 2010.

Edvardsson, D., Koch, S., and Nay, R. "Psychometric Evaluation of the English Language Person-Centred Climate Questionnaire—Patient Version." *Western Journal of Nursing Research*, 2009, *31*(2), 235–244.

Edvardsson, D., Koch, S., and Nay, R. "Psychometric Evaluation of the English Language Person-Centred Climate Questionnaire—Staff Version." *Journal of Nursing Management*, 2010, *18*(1), 54–60.

Frampton, S., and Guastello S. "Patient-Centered Care: More Than the Sum of Its Parts." *American Journal of Nursing*, 2010, *9*, 49–53.

Glickman, S. W., Boulding, W., Manary, M., Staelin, R., and others. "Patient Satisfaction and Its Relationship with Clinical Quality and Inpatient Mortality in Acute Myocardial Infarction." *Circulation Cardiovascular Quality and Outcomes*, 2010, *3*, 188–195.

Greene, J., and Hibbard, J. H. "Why Does Patient Activation Matter? An Examination of the Relationships Between Patient Activation and Health-Related Outcomes." *Journal of General Internal Medicine*, 2012, *27*(5), 520–526.

Healthcare Financial Management Association. "Patient Experience Scores Are Dragging Down VBP Scores." Sept. 21, 2010. HFMA. Accessed Sept. 10, 2012, at www.hfma.org/Publications/Leadership-Publication/Archives/E-Bulletins/2010/September/Patient-Experience-Scores-Are-Dragging-Down-VBP-Scores/

Institute of Medicine. *Crossing the Quality Chasm: A New Health System for the 21st Century*. Washington, DC: National Academy Press, 2001.

International Alliance of Patients' Organizations. "Declaration on Patient-Centred Healthcare." 2006, Accessed July 25, 2012, at www.patientsorganizations.org/declaration

Isaac, T., Zaslavsky, A. M., Cleary, P. D., and Landon, B. E. "The Relationship Between Patients' Perception of Care and Measures of Hospital Quality and Safety." *Health Services Research*, 2010, *45*, 1024–1040.

Neff, K. D. "Development and Validation of a Scale to Measure Self-Compassion." *Self and Identity*, 2003, *2*, 223–250.

Planetree, Inc., and Picker Institute. *Patient-Centered Care Improvement Guide*. Derby, CT, and Camden, ME: Planetree, Inc. and Picker Institute, 2008.

PART 2

Challenges and Solutions in Patient-Centered Care

3

Compassion in Action

Belinda Dewar and Susan B. Frampton

On the final morning of our annual mother-daughter weekend in 2010, my two sisters and I awoke to find that our mom had experienced a stroke during the night. We raced to the nearest hospital forty-five minutes away, and she was quickly moved into a cubicle in the Emergency Department, where tests, evaluations, and visits from nursing and medical staff began. My sisters and I remained by her side. We were an integral part of her care team, and the staff was supportive of that. My mom's eyes began to clear, as did her attention and ability to focus, although she was still unable to utter a word or respond to commands to blink her eyes. The CT scan came back positive for an embolic stroke, affecting the language center of her brain. The nursing staff was wonderful, speaking directly to my mom, noticing the nursing graduation necklace she wore and respectfully noting, "Oh, she's a nurse." I'm convinced my mother understood and appreciated this.

After several hours we moved upstairs to the neurology floor. We accompanied my mom's stretcher into the single-bed room, looked around at the clean, brightly painted walls and soothing artwork, surveyed the comfortable chairs for family and the window seat by the large picture window, and we all gave an audible sigh of relief. My sisters and I camped out for the next three days, taking shifts during the night, sleeping on the window seat that converted into a comfortable single bed. No one questioned our presence. We helped my mom to the bathroom, turned off the buzzer on her IV pole when she crimped her line with a bent elbow, got her ice cream when after two days on an IV she finally was able to eat pureed foods, took her for strolls around the unit when she regained enough strength and energy to get up and walk, read through all of the stroke education materials provided, and most important, wiped away her tears when she realized what had happened and what the challenges ahead were likely to be. My mom was discharged to home after a seventy-six-hour stay. It was a harrowing experience for all four of us, but what stands out in our memories several years later was the presence of caring, compassionate, competent caregivers.

I shared my family's experience months later with a group of nursing directors in a presentation at their annual patient-centered education day. After my talk, one of the women in the audience came up to speak with me to share her personal experience. She told me that her husband had had a serious stroke the previous year, and was admitted to the intensive care unit at a large academic medical center. But her experience was very different. Her voice trembling, she reported that the nursing staff forced her to leave for three-hour periods every three hours so that she wouldn't get in their way. "My husband died after four days in the ICU, and I missed half of his last hours on earth."

I have to believe that the nursing staff in that hospital was compassionate and that they probably did feel deep sympathy for a distressed wife whose husband lay dying in their intensive care unit, but they failed to take action to alleviate her suffering.
—Susan B. Frampton

DEFINING COMPASSION: The way in which we relate to other human beings when they are vulnerable. It has to be nurtured and supported. It involves noticing another person's vulnerability, experiencing an emotional reaction to this, and acting in some way with the person, in a way that is meaningful for people. It is defined by the people who give and receive it, and therefore interpersonal processes that capture what it means to people, are an important element of its promotion. (Dewar and Nolan, 2013)

Given this definition, it is interesting—disheartening even—that none of the definitions for patient-centered care presented earlier in this book include the term *compassion*. Perhaps, on some level, it is implied that patient-centered care must be delivered with compassion. However, recent events make it plain that compassion cannot be taken for granted as a baseline expectation for care. In the United Kingdom, revelations of an epidemic of uncompassionate care within the National Health Service (NHS) has caught the attention of health care policy leaders and the public alike, and inspired an outcry for reform. This lack of compassion is not exclusive to the NHS—far from it. A survey of eight hundred patients in the United States found that only 53 percent said that the health care system generally provides compassionate care (Lown, Rosen, and Marttila, 2011). And in a meeting with patient advocates in Africa about ways to improve health care quality in that region, a recurring theme was a pervasive culture of disrespect exhibited to patients and families by all caregivers, from physicians and nurses to housekeepers.

In this context, it bears stating explicitly: care delivered in the absence of compassion is *not patient-centered*. Compassionate action that supports the needs of the patient and family are the foundation of patient-centered care. Without action, there can be no real compassion. As fellow human beings, we know compassion when we see it, and we feel it acutely when it is lacking.

From Page to Practice

Take a moment to think about the concept of compassion in action, and of individuals who embody this ideal.

- Who comes to mind from the past and the present?
- What do these individuals have in common?
- What opportunities do you have to take compassionate action in your own life and work?

Interview your colleagues, family, and friends about their views on compassion in action and compare these to your own. What commonalities do you observe? Discuss ways that we can support one another to be more mindful of the opportunities to express compassion actively.

QUALITY OUTCOMES LINKED TO COMPASSION AND EMPATHY

From an altruistic perspective, the importance of compassion and empathy is obvious. Today, though, these characteristics of health care delivery have also become both a quality and business imperative given the links between a positive patient experience and better clinical and financial outcomes.

For example, Haslam (2007) reported in the *Medical Journal of Australia* that "patients have better treatment adherence and suffer from fewer major medical errors while under the care of empathetic doctors." Similarly, Rakel and others (2011) found that "empathy in the therapeutic encounter resulted in faster recovery times of flu patients." Hojat and colleagues (2011) reported that "health benefits were greater for diabetes patients (better cholesterol and blood-sugar scores) who were under the care of empathetic doctors."

The good news for caregivers is that compassion and empathy pay off in fewer malpractice claims. Virshup and others (1999) found that "physicians who are able to understand and appropriately respond to the emotional needs of their patients (act empathetically) are less likely to be hit with malpractice lawsuits." And for those to whom emotionally supportive behavior doesn't come naturally, research recently reported in *Hospital and Health Networks* found that "empathy seems to be a mutable trait. Certain conditions can blunt expressions of empathy and, conversely, certain awareness-building and reflection activities seem to be able to up-regulate empathic behavior" (Malloy and Otto, 2012). Compassionate actions and empathic responses can be taught.

COMPASSION AND EMPATHY IN PRACTICE

The Leadership in Compassionate Care Programme (LCCP) in Scotland has developed key processes and indicators that support embedding compassionate care in practice and education (Edinburgh Napier University and NHS Lothian, 2012). The program began in 2007 as an action research study that was underpinned by principles of appreciative inquiry and relationship-centered care. As part of this program, Dr. Belinda Dewar, a senior nurse, completed her PhD and identified, through in-depth exploration in one site, key processes and interpersonal characteristics required to develop knowledge to deliver compassionate relationship-centered care.

The approach to teaching and learning about acting compassionately with patients, families, and each other was based on the approach of appreciative inquiry (Dewar and Mackay, 2010). In this approach staff was supported to use observation and stories to help them to identify the aspects of their care that were compassionate, take a closer look to understand why these things happened, and explore how they could enable these practices to happen more of the time. Compassionate acts were not just observed and talked about with patients and families but with staff. It is important to ensure that caregivers feel safe and cared for so that they in turn can care for patients (Firth-Cozens and Cornwell, 2009). The centrality of the relationship in the act of compassionate caring is important. Von Dietze and Orb (2000) state: "Compassionate care becomes the moral way of treating the person because the person is more than just an individual. In times of illness or despair, words of advice or the simple caring presence of someone else who seeks to bring consolation, strength, hope, are given not because we are all individuals but because we are all part of the same humanity."

Through inquiring appreciatively, staff found out, for example, that patients, families, and staff valued:

- When staff went out of their way to shake a new relative's hand and ask them how they were, how they thought their relative was, and if they had any questions

- When staff took the time to ask questions about what mattered—finding out that a patient who was in her last few days of life preferred to lie on her right side

- When staff took the time to explain why the machine was bleeping

- When staff took the time to introduce the patient to other patients in the bay

- When staff offered patients hand-washing facilities after they had used the bedpan even if they had not wiped themselves

- When staff supported students not just to come alongside to watch a physical or technical procedure—but when they were invited to come alongside to watch some "difficult" or sensitive conversations

- When staff took the time to check out how each other was coping

- When staff listened to what mattered and went out of their way to try to provide this, even if this meant adapting existing policies

Many staff talked openly about how and why they did not always act in the ways identified above. However, rather than becoming defensive, staff questioned and subsequently changed their own practice. In so doing they showed a degree of humility and recognized that the "staff" do not always know what is best. Such insights helped them to develop a more questioning culture and a willingness to challenge taken-for-granted practices.

Adopting an appreciative approach highlighted the importance of such subtle interactions. Feeding this back to staff helped them to articulate, promote, and celebrate the skills involved in such practices. Some of this learning how to be compassionate in action is detailed in the following quotations.

> If someone wants to sit up—we know there are times when we think they should go to bed—but we need to listen to the patient and not just do things because they are convenient to us . . . there needs to be a bit of give and take, we need to talk this through. (Staff member)

> It has made us more aware of the bonding with the patient. You are not just showering a patient, you are using the opportunity to be with them, to talk to them about how they feel, to help them to feel less embarrassed about being naked in front of you. I think we are much more aware of this. We know more about the little things that matter to them and this is talked about more. (Staff member)

EMBEDDING COMPASSIONATE CARE IN EDUCATION

Such conversations represent an advanced and highly skillful form of relational practice that is nevertheless often not fully recognized, promoted, or celebrated within the culture that currently dominates health care. In other words this form of relational practice has not yet been recognized as a "core competency," nor has the need to promote experiential knowledge been fully valued.

Recognizing the importance of compassion as a core competency is something that is being developed in both education and practice in the wider LCCP in Scotland. Learnings from the wider program were integrated into the curriculum in a range of ways. For example, in a third-year module which teaches student nurses how to care for patients during the acute phase of illness, key elements that promote compassion were integrated into teaching and assessment (Adamson and Dewar, 2011). Although aspects of compassionate care were included within the scenarios in this module, the teaching team became aware that these elements were aware that using these elements was not explicit or assessed, making them appear more optional than a necessary requirement. Key elements that student nurses needed to consider that enabled care during the acute phase of illness to be not only safe and effective but also compassionate were made explicit and included:

- A deliberate welcome and a smile costs nothing

- Helping others to connect

- Knowing the little things that matter

- Being kept in the loop

- Being open and honest about expectations

These themes were developed both in the teaching and assessment of the module, where actor patients in the simulated environment would provide cues to prompt student nurses to demonstrate these processes. The themes represented the human connection often defined as "being with" the patient. The "being with" dimension of care requires more than technical expertise, and has been described as a form of responsive interaction where people require specific competences in order to deliver this (Schultz and others, 2007).

Supporting practitioners to develop the skills of compassion in caring involves helping them to notice and name these skills. By making these skills more explicit across educational environments and practice we can begin to value and celebrate them, as well as assess and monitor their existence.

A major challenge to the incorporation of such curriculum into both primary and continuing education for clinicians is a continuation of the traditional pattern of doctor-patient and nurse-patient relations, in which the appropriate or approved form of compassion is paternalistic benevolence at its best, and arrogant patronization at its worst. In many parts of the world, this old paradigm is alive and well, despite the demonstrated benefits of the newer, still-emerging pattern in which patients and their families and friends "are not so much subordinates of the authoritative doctor but more nearly partners" (Barber, 1976, p. 939).

PRACTICAL TOOLS TO ENHANCE COMPASSIONATE PRACTICE

Dewar and Nolan (2013) identifies that in order to deliver compassion we need to

1. Know who people are and what matters to them

2. Understand how they feel

3. Work together to shape the way things are done

Specific tools that help practitioners to engage with these processes are described here.

1. Know Who People Are and What Matters to Them

Knowing something about the person and what matters to them in a given situation, be it patient, family member, or staff member, is important if we are to respond appropriately to people's needs and enhance the care experience so that it feels compassionate for all involved. Staff decided to develop a set of key questions (see Table 3.1) that would help them explore what mattered to patients and families on a regular basis, and to find ways of sharing this information and debating its influence on care, more widely with the staff team.

Staff gained a great deal of information about the patient as a person and used this to influence care. In one situation, a patient who was blind was asked what was important to her. She replied, "Being read a chapter

Table 3.1 All About Me: Questions to Elicit Information About the Person to Enable Delivery of Compassion

What would you like staff to call you?

How would you feel if staff use terms like "darling," "love," "honey" when they speak to you?

Who are the people closest to you, and who do you want us to communicate with?

What are your thoughts and feelings about being in hospital?

What is your understanding of why you are in hospital?

Is there anything that is worrying you about being in hospital?

Is there anyone you would like to speak to? (doctor, chaplain, family member, friend, neighbor)

What is important to you while you are in hospital?

What support do you need from the people that care for you?

from the Bible, John:14." Staff realized there were no longer any Bibles in lockers. They had been removed some time ago, they understood because of equality and diversity issues and infection control. Staff tried to locate a Bible on neighboring wards and found nobody had one. They finally went to the Chaplaincy Centre and managed to retrieve one from a large storage cupboard full of Bibles. Following discussions with the chaplain, copies of Bibles and Korans were reinstated in all wards in the hospital. It would have been easy for staff to fall at the first hurdle with this example, but they persevered.

Staff did worry that they would not always be able to provide the aspects that patients felt were important to them, making them feel that asking the question in the first instance involved taking a risk. It could feel safer not to ask. However, this example demonstrated that the organization could be challenged, based on powerful knowledge, which was person knowledge. Working as a team to deliver on this, and persevering, were key attributes contributing to a successful outcome.

Asking questions such as those in Table 3.1 is about a skilled interaction. Staff recognized that questions could not be seen as a set framework to be "ticked off" and signed as completed. Rather, questions had to be asked with sensitivity and thoughtfulness, and this happened over a period of time, rather than as a one-time activity. Staff members could not always make links between what they had learned about what mattered to people and how this influenced caregiving. It seemed easy, for example, if a patient said that it was important to have a daily newspaper, to provide this. It was perhaps more difficult when a patient said that what was important to them was not to upset people, for staff to reflect on how this influenced care they might deliver. Thus, information did not always relate specifically to a care task but to the way in which people developed relationships.

From Page to Practice

Take a moment to reflect on the following questions:

- How do you get to know the patient as a person?
- What questions do you ask them?
- How do you share this information with others to help them to use this knowledge to influence the way care is delivered?

---

2. Understand How They Feel

Understanding a person's unique experience is important to enable compassion to be realized in practice. Using emotional touchpoints can help us to tap into the experience of the person. The technique is essentially about understanding how people *feel* about their experience through the vehicle of storytelling. The method focuses on emotion by asking patients and their families to think about key points in the care journey and to select from a range of emotional words those that best describe how they felt about an experience (Dewar and others, 2010).

A touchpoint is a point in the experience such as "coming into the hospital," "getting information," "visiting times," and so forth. The person who is sharing an experience identifies a touchpoint and is asked to say how he or she feels about this. To help express the feelings, the person is shown a range of emotional words and asked to select those that sum up what the experience meant in regard to the touchpoint. These words could be negative, such as "lost" or "embarrassed," or positive, for example, "relieved" or "safe." The storyteller is asked why he or she felt that way, and these feelings about the experience are written down and the story is fed back to the person soon after the conversation to check for accuracy. The story, which can be anonymized, is then shared with others as a stimulus for learning about excellent care practices and those that need to be developed further.

Thus, this process of doing emotional touchpoints enables people to enter into a dialogue where there is less emphasis on what is right or wrong or good or bad, but rather staff, patients, and families are encouraged to relive happenings, express their perceptions, feelings, assumptions, regrets, and wishes with the purpose of developing understanding, rather than finding fault or making judgments.

The example below of a relative's experience of "being around" when his mother was taken to the toilet shows the range of emotional words that summed up the experience for him:

- Emotional touchpoint: Going to the toilet
- Emotional words selected: *irritated and misunderstood, belittled, proud*

With a few staff, they need to develop their communication skills. On these occasions I felt irritated and misunderstood. I asked a nurse if she could help Mum get to the loo. The nurse said yes and asked if I wanted to help her—to which I said yes, as I had done this at home. What I was expecting was to take her into the loo, let her sit down and shut the door while I wait outside. The nurse brought a commode to the bedside, stood her up and took down her pants in front of me. I think my Mum felt belittled. I just accepted that it had happened and did not say anything. There were so many examples of good communication though from domestics, nurses and doctors—the whole team. My Mum needed the loo and I told somebody—they said this was not a problem and asked me to wait outside. I could hear them outside the room and they were chatting away to Mum at her level—they were having a laugh together and sharing things. I felt proud as the staff had probably heard what she was saying so many times already but they reacted as if they had heard what she was saying for the first time. This felt good. (Relative story)

The key learning identified by staff related to the challenge of helping people to speak out when they were upset about something and the real skill of "being with" a person with a cognitive impairment and sharing these skills with others. We can see that even where a negative feeling was expressed this did not always mean that there was a deficiency in the service, but rather there was misunderstanding about the staff's intention, which led to a negative experience for the relative. It is important to note, however, that supporting staff to see the balance in the story needed careful facilitation.

Also evident here is that this method helped us to tap into positive experiences of caring that often remain hidden as they are not easy to articulate. Listening to a person with dementia repeating a story as if you have heard it for the first time is an expert skill that would not have been recognized by the nurses on the ward as something they do well.

NHS Education Scotland and The Leadership in Compassionate Care Programme at Edinburgh Napier University and NHS Lothian have produced an excellent resource in the form of a DVD that introduces the method of emotional touchpoints. (You can access this learning resource at: www.knowledge.scot.nhs.uk/making-a-difference/making-a-difference/valuing-feedback.aspx.)

3. Working Together to Shape the Way Things Are Done

How we work together and use the knowledge about what matters to people and how they feel can require skilled interaction, which can be difficult to describe precisely to others. Sometimes compassionate actions are not accessible to our consciousness. Think about, for example, a member of staff saying that she always welcomes people to the ward. She may not be fully aware what she actually does. After observing her in practice we realize that she:

- Was really busy but took the time to stop what she was doing and make eye contact with new visitors and ask if she could help them

- Walked with them to where their relative was in the ward and used this opportunity to talk to them along the way by asking some specific questions

- Appeared calm and unhurried when she was speaking

- Asked such questions as "How are you?" and "Have you any questions?" and conveying, "I will be able to come back and speak to you in about half an hour"

Making observations about what is going on and how people are interacting (for example, during meal times, how these are organized, where people sit, how people are given choice, how people are helped to eat, and so on) can help people to understand the subtle aspects of their interpersonal communication that enhance compassionate caring.

Interaction between people is rarely the focus of systematic observation and audit in health care yet it is at the heart of compassionate care. Healthcare Improvement Scotland, working with The Leadership in Compassionate Care Team, has developed a tool which can be used to observe and feedback on interaction (see healthcareimprovementscotland.org/programmes/inspecting_and_regulating_care/caring_for_older_people/procedures_and_tools/observation_tool.aspx?theme=mobile). With this tool, interaction is observed over a 20-minute period and categorized into positive, neutral, or negative interactions.

Examples of the type of interaction in each category are shown in Table 3.2.

Staff receive feedback about the way they interact and are supported to reflect on this and consider future development of practice.

All of these processes help us to gain feedback on aspects of care that are compassionate. By using the processes identified above the concept of compassion can be articulated and actions that enable it to be realized can be cocreated with staff, patients, and families so that they are meaningful. Some examples of compassionate actions that resulted from using the feedback processes highlighted in Table 3.2 included:

- Noticing a person liked to wear makeup and continuing to do this for her when she could not do this herself
- Introducing patients to other patients on the ward
- Asking family if and how they want to be involved in care
- Asking people how they feel about their experience
- Adapting practices to meet individual needs, such as carefully assessing the appropriateness of two hourly turns for a person in the very last stages of their life
- Making sure we tell people what they specifically have done well

PUTTING COMPASSION FIRST

Compassion occurs at a deeply personal level, person to person. However, when organizations reorganize standard processes and structures to put compassion first, the results—as demonstrated in the two field examples that follow—can be extraordinary.

Table 3.2 Examples of Positive, Neutral, and Negative Interactions

Positive Interaction	Neutral Interaction	Negative Interaction
• Showing interest in and knowledge of the patient as a person • Assessing information needs, tailoring information to the individual, and checking understanding • Giving options, seeking preferences, and respecting choices • Encouraging the "person" during care tasks and recognizing individual achievements • Welcoming patients and visitors onto the ward • Responding warmly to their questions • Recognizing and responding to their concerns and emotions	• Speaking to someone in a manner that lacks empathy but is not necessarily rude or disrespectful • Explaining what is going to happen without offering choice or the opportunity to ask questions • Not taking an active interest in what the person is saying and with no engagement beyond minimal response giving • Offering brief verbal explanations and some encouragement, but only that necessary to complete the care task • Not recognizing their underlying concerns and emotions	• Ignoring or talking over someone during conversations • Telling someone to wait for something without any explanation or comfort • Telling someone they can't have something without good reason or explanation • Telling or instructing a person to do something without explanation, discussion, or offering assistance • Treating a person in a childlike or disapproving way • Using childlike language or "elder speak" • Not allowing a person to use their abilities or make choices (even if said with "kindness") • Seeking choice but then ignoring or overruling it • Being rude, short, or unfriendly

FIELD EXAMPLE: **EASING CHILD AND FAMILY EMOTIONAL DISTRESS IN LUMBAR PUNCTURES**

Royal Children's Hospital, Melbourne, Australia

At The Royal Children's Hospital in Melbourne, Australia, children with cancer need to have regular tests where bone marrow and spinal fluid are removed by inserting needles into the pelvic bone and into the spinal column. These procedures need to be repeated many times on each child, sometimes up to forty times during two years of treatment. Traditionally, the procedures have been painful, and many children found them distressing or terrifying. The level of sedation was often unsatisfactory. Parents described their children becoming anxious days before each procedure was due. For the past twelve years, a team led by Dr. Catherine Crock has worked to change this by improving partnerships with the patients and families. The medical staff worked closely with the parents to identify problems and seek solutions; many changes were made. This has led to a service where families say they feel safe and secure when they come to the operating theatre for their child's procedure.

The patient-centered approach has been developed and implemented in partnership with families at every stage. The aim is for children to go to sleep calmly and wake up happily. To assist with this, theatre scheduling has been redesigned to suit the families, not the hospital. Families arrive as little as 30 minutes before the time of their procedure. A music therapist is present and plays with the children. The child stays fully dressed in street clothes and can play games on an iPad or listen to specially composed *HUSH* music (www.hush.org.au) while going to sleep. They have their choice of ten flavors (such as cola or chocolate) to put in the gas masks. Children can choose whether to go to sleep quickly or slowly, on their parent's knee or on the bed. They may elect not to have a mask and have an intravenous injection via a vein to which numbing cream has been applied. They may prefer to talk to the anesthetic

(Continued)

technician about football or even sing their team's theme song. Parents are supported by an extra person, and given a hug or reassurance after their child is asleep. Parents are invited into the recovery room before their child is awake so that the child wakes up to the comforting of their parents. The child leaves the theatre with his or her parents a total time after arrival of perhaps an hour.

Redesigning the service from a patient-centered viewpoint has led to quite startling results. The most obvious is the change in the children themselves, with several children commenting that their favorite part of hospital visits is having their lumbar punctures! Less obvious but equally important has been the change on the health professionals themselves. Developing a culture of respect for families has also nurtured a culture of respect between the staff. Each member of the team is prepared to take the time to figure out what approach works best for each patient and family. Each member of the team trusts and looks after other team members as they work. Quick review sessions are held with parents to check that the plan for their child is working, and with other team members to confirm that all is going well. Job satisfaction has soared.

One mother, Jen, describes how her eight-year-old son, Josh, has benefited from this approach. "The presence of compassion in the operating theatre has significantly reduced the stress and fear associated with having a child . . . my child . . . my Josh, diagnosed with a life-threatening medical condition. The empathy shown by the theatre team, and their encouragement for parents to be involved in the decision making, has allowed me to experience some positivity and to feel useful, rather than hopeless or helpless—even in the face of the most pronounced pain and fear I have ever experienced." She goes on to add, "The greatest gift they bestowed on me, however, is that they have made Josh feel protected and secure. When Josh is feeling scared and vulnerable he is anxious and unhappy—which adversely affects his health and treatment. But Josh has very quickly learned that he can trust Catherine, and the adults around her, and he has become resilient, brave, and empowered."

FIELD EXAMPLE: **TAKING THE STING OUT OF THE LAB**

Sharp Coronado Hospital, Coronado, California, USA

The Sharp Coronado Hospital laboratory team goes above and beyond their duties by creating exceptional experiences for patients and a uniquely positive culture within the laboratory department. Certainly, it is not one of life's most pleasant experiences to have one's blood drawn. However, this team has come up with innovative ways to make the process better and less painful for patients, and in so doing improved their work lives and team spirit. When patients enter the lab, they are invited to unwind in a designated patient lounge before their appointments. The team advocated for turning the lounge into a spa-like environment, where soft music, lovely works of art, and the aroma of lavender have a calming effect. As the person is escorted from the lounge to the drawing area, the experience continues to surprise and delight. Phlebotomists begin by providing hand massages to patients during their blood draw as a soothing way to increase blood flow, release tension, and help reduce stress and anxiety. With patient-centered care in mind, team members offer gentle encouragement during the procedure because tender touching promotes a deeper sense of connection and a feeling of being cared for. As patients leave to reenter the lobby they are offered spa water and fruit as appropriate.

In addition to incorporating human touch and complementary modalities into their practice, the lab technicians went one step further by launching a unique, personalized service called "drive-through phlebotomy." This simple and thoughtful innovation was devised when the lab team realized that many community residents required frequent blood draws but had limited mobility or difficulty getting dressed. After caring for many of these elderly patients, and seeing how inconvenient it was for them and their caregivers to come into the lab, the team launched the new system for the patients and their families. A call to the laboratory prior to

(Continued)

arriving at the hospital allows a phlebotomist to meet eligible patients curbside, either in front of the hospital or next to the Emergency Department. This service reduces wait times and fall risks while appreciably improving comfort.

A bulletin board boasts notes from grateful patients, and it is updated weekly to display positive feedback. The department's overall patient satisfaction score from February 2011 to March 2012 is at the 82nd percentile. In addition, lab employee satisfaction is at an all-time high, and turnover is at an all-time low.

CONCLUSION: COMPASSION AND TRANSFORMATION

Each of us holds within us the potential to do something extraordinary. Today in health care, it's not the rocket science of the next medical breakthrough or ever more sophisticated technology that's extraordinary—that has become our stock in trade. What's become much rarer is simple kindness and compassion in action, which the early patient-centered pioneers understood so well and practiced generously. This book is dedicated to one of those early pioneers, Laura Gilpin, who embodied compassion in action.

Laura was a night nurse on the very first Planetree hospital unit in the 1980s, and she dedicated her life to promoting the importance of kindness and caring in health care. She was a night nurse for several reasons, in part because she didn't like to inflict pain even in the service of healing and there are less treatments and injections required on the night shift, and in part because she realized that her job as a caregiver was to create an environment that truly supported healing. At night on her unit she was a sleep vigilante, and used to say that her job was to protect the sleep of her patients, because sleep was healing. What a simple kindness, and yet extraordinarily difficult to achieve in today's fast-paced, high-tech, high-stress environment. In many ways this example is the essence of the challenge of compassion in action and of true patient-centered care: how do we infuse kindness and consideration into the work that we do, every day, for every patient? This is a transformational opportunity and the challenge before us regardless of where we find ourselves in the world.

REFERENCES

Adamson, L., and Dewar, B. "Compassion in the Nursing Curriculum: Making It More Explicit." *Journal of Holistic Healthcare*, 2011, *8*(3), 42–45.

Barber, B. "Seminars in Medicine of the Beth Israel Hospital, Boston. Compassion in Medicine: Toward New Definitions and New Institutions." *New England Journal of Medicine*, 1976, *295*(17), 939–943.

Dewar, B., and Mackay, R. "Appreciating Compassionate Care in Acute Care Setting Caring for Older People." *International Journal of Older People Nursing*, 2010, *5*, 299–308.

Dewar, B., Mackay, R., Smith S, Pullin, S., and Tocher, R. "Use of Emotional Touchpoints as a Method of Tapping into the Experience of Receiving Compassionate Care in a Hospital Setting." *Journal of Nursing Research*, 2010, *15*(1), 29–41.

Dewar, B., and Nolan, M. "Caring About Caring: Developing a Model to Implement Compassionate Relationship Centred Care in an Older People Care Setting." *International Journal of Nursing Studies*, 2013, doi:10:1016\j.ijnurstu2013.01.008

Edinburgh Napier University and NHS Lothian. "Leadership in Compassionate Care Programme, Final Report." Edinburgh: Edinburgh Napier University, 2012.

Firth-Cozens, J., and Cornwell, J. *The Point of Care: Enabling Compassionate Care in Acute Hospital Settings*. London: Kings Fund, 2009.

Haslam, N. "Humanizing Medical Practice: The Role of Empathy." *Medical Journal of Australia*, 2007, *187*(7), 381–382.

Hojat, M., Louis, D. Z., Markham, F. W., Wender, R., and others. "Physicians' Empathy and Clinical Outcomes for Diabetic Patients." *Academic Medicine*, 2011, *86*(3), 359–364.

Lown, B. A., Rosen, J., and Marttila, J. "An Agenda for Improving Compassionate Care: A Survey Shows About Half of Patients Say Such Care Is Missing." *Health Affairs*, 2011, *30*(9), 1772–1778.

Malloy, R., and Otto, J. "A Steady Dose of Empathy." *Hospital and Health Networks Daily*, June 7, 2012.

Rakel, D., Barrett, B., Zhang, Z., Hoeft, T., and others. "Perception of Empathy in the Therapeutic Encounter: Effects on the Common Cold." *Patient Education and Counseling*, 2011, *85*(3), 390–397.

Schultz, R., Hebert, R. S., Dew, M. A., Brown, S. L., and others. "Patient Suffering and Caregiver Compassion: New Opportunities for Research, Practice, and Policy." *Gerontologist*, 2007, *47*(1), 4–13.

Virshup, B. B., Oppenberg, A. A., and Coleman, M. M. "Strategic Risk Management: Reducing Malpractice Claims Through More Effective Patient-Doctor Communication. *American Journal of Medical Quality*, 1999, *14*(4), 153–159.

Von Dietze, E., and Orb, A. "Compassionate Care: A Moral Dimension of Nursing." *Nursing Inquiry*, 2000, *7*(3), 166–174.

4

Words That Work: Patient-Centered Physician Communication

Dorothea Wild

Three medical residents and a couple of medical students exchange conspiratorial glances as they wait for me to lead them into Mrs. P's room. They know I'm likely to talk about "effective counseling," one of the goals for this month-long internal medicine rotation. They also know that counseling Mrs. P. won't be easy. At fifty-four years old, she cycles in and out of the hospital for lung problems—asthma combined with the effects of uncontrolled smoking. Now Mrs. P. is nearly ready to go home. Our team faces the dreaded specter: how to plan her discharge. The team seems convinced that in a matter of weeks or months, her smoking will land her back here again.

As we stand in the hallway, I ask the intern who follows Mrs. P. to tell me what he knows about the patient's feelings about her smoking. The intern seems flustered. "She doesn't want to quit," he replies. I ask again, gently, "But what does Mrs. P. think about her smoking?" The team is silent. They seem to be thinking about my question—and the assumption underneath the question that it's very important what Mrs. P thinks. There is some thoughtful silence around

91

me. My guess is that "counseling" so far has consisted of telling Mrs. P.: "You really need to stop smoking." Perhaps the intern has shown kindness; perhaps, irritation. But from our baseline assessment of incoming interns, I suspect that the intern had done more talking than listening.

I ask the intern: "What was your opening question for the conversation?" My implicit message is this: most counseling, and most interactions in general, should start with a question—and certainly not with a lecture. More silence. I tell the intern that when we enter Mrs. P.'s room, we'll see how a more patient-centered conversation might work. The intern will lead the conversation, and the rest of us will support him. I also suggest how to get things started: "Mrs. P., I would like to talk with you about your smoking." And then he should ask: "Is that okay?" After that, I tell him to follow the patient's lead and use active listening techniques he has practiced in a classroom before—silence, nonverbal encouragements to keep talking (uh-huh), and repeating some of the phrases. That is, I want the intern to pay attention to where the patient leads the conversation and to respond to what she says, rather than following a scripted interchange.

As instructed, the intern greets Mrs. P., (re)introduces himself and the team, and asks if we can speak with her for a few minutes about her smoking. The patient rolls her eyes and says "Okay . . . I guess." She sighs ostentatiously. The intern seems unsure how to deal with the eye-rolling and the sigh. When the patient does not say anything, the intern moves into lecture mode. Mrs. P. turns her face toward the window. I wait about thirty seconds before I interject, "Mrs. P., I noticed that you were rolling your eyes when Dr. Smith asked you if he could talk to you about smoking. . . ." Mrs. P. bursts out: "I am sick of you all coming in here on your high horse and telling me I shouldn't smoke. Do you think I don't know that? Do you think I'm an idiot? Of course I know it's bad, especially with my asthma. But you don't know what my life is like."

Mrs. P. has broken her silence, and the intern now sees how to keep the conversation alive. He nods as he listens to Mrs. P. describe *how stressful she finds her work. As an animal control officer for the city, she sees dogs and cats and even horses that have come close to death from neglect or from horrible acts of cruelty. Mrs. P. says that she doesn't even like to smoke, and she knows what it does to her lungs, but it's the only thing that really helps her relax. She isn't about to quit the job, either. The animals need her, and she needs the income.*

While the rest of the team use body language to convey that they are sympathetic and attentive, the intern continues the conversation. He asks Mrs. P. if she has any ideas for how she might quit smoking. Mrs. P. says she has heard of smokeless cigarettes (a nicotine inhaler) and wonders if they might help. She knows a bit about pharmacologic options for quitting, and she asks questions about how medication might help.

In less than five minutes, the atmosphere in the room has shifted from contentious to supportive. The woman who had been a non-cooperative carrier of disease has become visible as a person. Now she and the team are working toward a common goal rather than annoying one another. We compliment Mrs. P. about her good ideas and tell her that the intern will return with information about nicotine inhalers and about medications that support smoking cessation.

—Dorothea Wild

In reflecting on my own residency training (in the late 1990s in the institution where I now practice), I recognize how training has changed since then. When I was an intern, we knew we were supposed to be caring. But what exactly did caring sound like? And was communicating that I cared as important as mastering statistical principles and understanding evidence-based medicine, topics that dominated textbooks? Had anyone talked to us about how to show caring when we were tired, hungry, and behind schedule? I had never had trouble caring. What had been difficult was learning how to express my caring: how to use conversation to connect to patients; how to empower people to change their behavior rather than ranting; and most of all how to accomplish it all within a normal admission timeline, rather than during a leisurely conversation.

I know that some people object to repeating lines that are scripted, that they balk at being told what to say. But I would have been very grateful to anybody who gave me those opening lines: "I would like to talk about your smoking. Is that okay?" (And obviously, somebody finally did.)

My colleagues and I want to help the next generation come by this knowledge sooner and more easily. And so, we created an environment for our trainees that would give them the words, and the skills, so that even at 2:00 a.m., confronted by an angry patient, working on their eighth admission of the night, they could tap into a repertoire of questions and responses that would allow a patient to feel heard.

That journey is still ongoing and far from over, but I would like to describe our progress so far. My hope is to show the power of teaching scripts to physicians and to show that by weaving such teaching into a tapestry that also incorporates role modeling, detailed feedback, and constant evaluation, we can improve the way physicians talk, and change how they listen.

TRANSFORMING AN ORGANIZATION'S COMMUNICATION CURRICULUM: STEP BY STEP

Our institution aimed to transform the entire communication curriculum. The transformation consisted of:

A. Increasing problem awareness and obtaining baseline data

B. Designing the training content and planning how to teach it

C. Addressing the hidden curriculum and training faculty role models

D. Implementing processes that enable and support caring

E. Evaluation

A. Increasing Problem Awareness and Obtaining Baseline Data

People will only change if they are aware of a problem. Decision makers and potential allies can be made aware of a problem with communication if they are offered a combination of anecdotes and objective data. Gathering data before attempting to make any change is also important, both to make a case when asking for resources, and also to assess changes later. In our case, we had a retreat with the CEO where we shared our anecdotes, and talked about the strategic value of integrating Planetree as a teaching philosophy into the residency training. We felt that developing a curriculum and validating it would not just help our patients (and improve satisfaction scores), but also provide data, research opportunities, an opportunity to distinguish our institution from other teaching hospitals, and help in recruiting new physicians. We used two surveys for baseline data: a published survey to assess the hidden curriculum and a revised existing survey that addressed faculty teaching behaviors.

From Page to Practice

Use this survey to obtain baseline data about your organization's current state.

Faculty Teaching Skills Survey

Please evaluate each of the following attendings based on your overall experience with them throughout the past year. (1 = strongly agree; 2 = agree; 3 = undecided; 4 = disagree; 5 = strongly disagree; N/A = not applicable)

(Continued)

	Faculty 1	Faculty 2	Faculty 3
Learning climate	☺ ☹ ☒	☺ ☹ ☒	☺ ☹ ☒
1. Made learner feel comfortable asking questions on rounds	1 2 3 4 5 n/a	1 2 3 4 5 n/a	1 2 3 4 5 n/a
2. Assessed the needs of the learner	1 2 3 4 5 n/a	1 2 3 4 5 n/a	1 2 3 4 5 n/a
3. Expressed respect for learner	1 2 3 4 5 n/a	1 2 3 4 5 n/a	1 2 3 4 5 n/a
4. Was a good role model of a caring doctor	1 2 3 4 5 n/a	1 2 3 4 5 n/a	1 2 3 4 5 n/a
5. Avoided sexism and racism	1 2 3 4 5 n/a	1 2 3 4 5 n/a	1 2 3 4 5 n/a
Communication of goals			
6. Stated goals and expectations of the team	1 2 3 4 5 n/a	1 2 3 4 5 n/a	1 2 3 4 5 n/a
Patient-centered care			
7. Communicated care, concern, and interest in the patient as a person	1 2 3 4 5 n/a	1 2 3 4 5 n/a	1 2 3 4 5 n/a
8. Explored emotional aspects of patient's illnesses	1 2 3 4 5 n/a	1 2 3 4 5 n/a	1 2 3 4 5 n/a
Evaluation			
9. Asked learners to discuss differential diagnosis on most patients	1 2 3 4 5 n/a	1 2 3 4 5 n/a	1 2 3 4 5 n/a
Feedback			
10. Gave learners regular, useful feedback on their performance	1 2 3 4 5 n/a	1 2 3 4 5 n/a	1 2 3 4 5 n/a
Self-directed learning			
11. Encouraged learners to pursue the literature to answer specific questions	1 2 3 4 5 n/a	1 2 3 4 5 n/a	1 2 3 4 5 n/a

Standardized Patients and OSCEs   We also started videotaping our residents' interactions with real patients and standardized patients. The standardized patients were used as a form of Objective Structured Clinical Examination (OSCE). They usually describe a communication challenge, such as counseling for tobacco cessation in a disinterested patient, and are scored with a validated score card. From all these sources, we were able to paint a convincing picture to ourselves, to the hospital's administration, and to external funders: our everyday behavior was not living up to our Planetree philosophy, and we wanted to do something about it.

B. Designing the Training Content and Planning How to Teach It

The curriculum we designed mixes general communication training with training on how to approach particular populations. We also realized that we needed to do more to teach communication than to design a lecture series around it. So we experimented with ways to integrate communication teaching into ANY teaching or clinical encounter. As an example, we developed "two-minute teaching techniques" to integrate communication training into our teaching rounds (see Table 4.1).

Of particular importance for us was to organize the teaching, assessment, and faculty development around a common evaluation structure. We used an abridged version of the Calgary-Cambridge Observation Guide (available at www.skillscascade.com/handouts/CalgaryCambridge Guide.pdf). We chose this assessment because it was suitable for scoring our six-minute standardized patient encounters. We also found it worked to plan lectures, structure feedback, and standardize faculty teaching assessment. For example, in our faculty sessions, we would watch a faculty member as he or she interacted with a standardized patient. Each faculty member would score this encounter individually. Then we compared our assessments. This was a very easy way to bring to the surface different approaches to various communication tasks. It also helped us reach an agreement on behavioral definitions of patient-centered communication, such as what empathy looked like. These behavioral discussions, in turn, made it much easier to teach communication skills during rounds.

Table 4.1 Short Teaching Pearls to Integrate Communication Teaching into Teaching Encounters

A Let the resident ask "what else?" three times

Share the example below (Barrier, 2003). Then have the resident ask "what else?" three times at the next encounter.

Physician-Centered	**Patient-Centered**
Physician: What brings you here today?	Physician: What brings you here today?
Patient: I have headaches.	Patient: I have headaches.
Physician: Where are the headaches? How long do they last? What do you do to relieve them?	Physician: What else?
	Patient: Well, I have problems sleeping.
	Physician: What else?
	Patient: I am very worried about my son. He is using drugs.

B Ask for Patient Teach-Back of Admission Diagnosis

For an admitted patient: Ask the residents outside the patient's room if they have explained the admission diagnosis to the patient. Residents usually will say yes. When in the room, ask the patient: "Mr. Jones, what did you understand about what brings you into the hospital?" If the patient knows exactly what the presumptive diagnosis is, compliment the admitting team. If the answer is, "I don't know," have the resident explain again. This technique gives the teacher the opportunity to amplify the plan for the patient, and role model for the group how to communicate. Afterward, ask the group for feedback for the resident and provide feedback yourself.

C Explain the Plan of the Day

End each patient encounter in rounds with asking the intern or medical student: "Can you explain the plan of the day to your patient?" Again, gently correct jargon if it occurs, and review what interests most patients (actionable information, possible discomfort with procedures) and what does not interest most of them (pathophysiologic explanations of how particular investigations work.)

Table 4.1 (*Continued*)

D Identify Empathetic Opportunities

Observe a learner interacting with a patient for five minutes. Ask the learner afterward to reflect on the presence of empathetic opportunities (can also be done with a group of learners.) For more advanced learners, ask them to respond to the empathic opportunity following the NURS acronym: Name the emotion; express Understanding; express Respect for the patient, and voice your Support (Fortin, Dwamena, Frankel, and Smith, 2012).

E Review Ask Me 3

Ask in rounds: "When time is short, what are the most important things to tell patients?" Then review the Ask Me 3 technique (National Patient Safety Foundation):

1. What is my main problem?
2. What do I need to do?
3. Why is it important for me to do this?

Observe resident teach the patient this technique and then answer the three questions. Again, comment on jargon, active listening, and response to empathetic opportunities.

F Questions to Start a Counseling Session

Observe resident perform a patient counseling. Either before or after, ask him or her to (1) start with, "Is it okay if we talk about xxx?" and (2) use active listening techniques for the first two minutes of the conversation. Have learners reflect on the differences between the two conversations.

Finally, we had to make sure to look at our outcomes. For this purpose, we designed a set of biannual OSCE scenarios, where we taped all our learners and core faculty using two or three communication stations. Examples for stations include breaking bad news, interacting with a patient with low health literacy, and admitting to a medical mistake. The communication situations came either from real incidents in the hospital, or from the literature. We shortened the scenarios so they could be done within six minutes, and scored them with a validated score card. We also used a burnout assessment tool, and sought feedback from our nurses and patients.

From Page to Practice

Trial the OSCE scenario below, tape it, and score it with your peers using the Calgary-Cambridge Observation Guide, found at www.skillscascade. com/handouts/CalgaryCambridgeGuide.pdf.

Patient Scenario

Your name is John Finch and you are forty-five years old. You have only completed elementary school. You work as a custodian. You have never learned to read properly, and have a lot of trouble reading and understanding written information. You are embarrassed about this and pretend that you can understand written instructions. If somebody asks you to read something to them, you pretend that you forgot your reading glasses.

You were recently hospitalized for chest pain and are now seeing your primary care physician for follow-up. Before the hospitalization, you were not taking any medications. You were hospitalized overnight and discharged on a baby aspirin with written discharge instructions. You have no idea what they say.

You are here today to discuss your hospitalization and your cholesterol results. Your cholesterol is high, and you will need to be started on a new medication.

Allow the doc to explain your test results without jumping in too much. Indicate subtly that you don't understand some things (for example, look down at the floor whenever the resident uses jargon; if asked if you have any questions, answer, "Whatever you say, doc"). Make at least one incorrect statement about your cholesterol and the plan (such as, "Should I take more cholesterol pills if I eat something fatty?").

Resident Script

You are in the clinic and about to see Mr. Finch as a follow-up visit. Mr. Finch was recently in the hospital for chest pain. The patient was ruled out for an ACS, but his LDL is 189. He needs to be started on a statin. As you review the chart, you notice that the patient has only completed elementary school, and that he works as a custodian.

Your goals for the next six minutes are:

1. Assess the patient's understanding of his hospital discharge instructions
2. Discuss the patient's need for the new medicine
3. Discuss any possible side effects.

Be sure to assess the patient's understanding of your instructions!
In the interest of time, do not discuss diet.

C. Addressing the Hidden Curriculum and Training Role Models

One of the central challenges in teaching patient-centered communication is to recognize the hidden curriculum—that is, the implicit teaching of values and behavior norms that takes place through examples, stories, and daily interactions (Haidet and others, 2005). The hidden curriculum is the main determinant for how physicians learn what are acceptable behaviors and values. To address the hidden curriculum, we needed to make sure that the faculty were effective role models. We recruited an outside faculty member to meet with a group of core faculty once a month. This gave us a forum for sharing experiences, reflecting on our efforts, reviewing each other's tapes of patients, and supporting each other. We also used this time to score resident tapes together, review curricular content, and discuss methods for providing effective feedback. With the help of grant support, we were able to invite high-level speakers for grand rounds. These lectures demonstrated the evidence behind various communication techniques, provided more academic role models for our residents, gave us teaching pearls for morning report, and made it more acceptable in rounds and other forums to discuss techniques of patient counseling, or research around communication.

We were inspired by the literature from Inui and colleagues about changing the culture at Indiana University School of Medicine to try and influence our institution in other ways. Inui and colleagues had posited that although cultural change can't be forced, culture is shaped and sustained by multiple every day encounters. Changing some of these daily encounters will therefore change culture. His group has also described how culture change can be fostered by a principle of recognizing and disseminating success (Cottingham and others, 2008). When attention is focused not only on the problems and deficiencies, but also on the successes and on resources already present in an institution, the motivation for change grows much more quickly.

One way of fostering attention to successes and strengths is called appreciative inquiry. An appreciative inquiry is a technique to spend time reviewing a positive experience to learn how the experience happened and how it could be repeated. In keeping with this approach, we chose to start our faculty development sessions with sharing one story about an encounter that went well, and reflecting together on the root causes of this success, and considering how we might make it happen more often.

Finally, as a group we reviewed the biannual OSCE tapes and discussed how to teach the competencies we were hoping to foster. This led us to emphasize the value of taking residents with us when conducting family conferences, and it helped us discover time-efficient new ways to observe residents communicating. It also led us to form pairs of faculty who would observe and (tactfully) critique each other as we taught residents or interacted with patients. Comments from our colleagues provided opportunities for reflection.

From Page to Practice

Initiate an appreciative debrief. In a meeting, identify an incident in the recent past where things went well. With the group, reflect on (1) who was involved, (2) exactly what happened, (3) what resources, people, constellations made this successful event happen, and (4) whether an event like this could happen more often.

D. Implementing Processes That Support Caring

A fundamental tenet of patient-centered care is that caring for the patient will not work without caring for the caregiver as well. In our case, that meant to build relationships which would allow for open and honest feedback, and to change structures that were impeding good relationships with patients. Measures we took to foster relationships included the appreciative debriefs described above, forming peer-mentoring teams among residents and among faculty, and augmenting our monthly faculty development meetings with weekly check-ins among ourselves. We added exercises to foster reflections and self-awareness to the monthly ethics lecture for our residents. All incoming employed physicians participate in a Planetree retreat in which they work and bond with each other and employees from all over the institution. During this retreat, the incoming resident group has a four-hour coaching session with standardized patients to practice patient-centered communication.

E. Evaluation

We used many instruments to measure change. Among them are resident surveys to measure burnout, nurses' surveys about physician communication behavior, tracking the class score in the OSCEs, self-assessment by faculty of their comfort with teaching, and surveys to detect changes in the hidden curriculum and faculty teaching behavior survey. We also developed and implemented an objective structured teaching evaluation (OSTE.) An OSTE features a standardized learner, rather than a patient; in our case this was a medical student in trouble. This exercise brought out how differently faculty approached counseling and feedback. Seeing how differently the residents handled the exercise also led us to become much more involved with how residents provide feedback to their interns and medical students.

HOW THE CHANGE AFFECTED PATIENT AND STAFF EXPERIENCE

In our repeat surveys, residents rated faculty higher in domains such as providing feedback and responding to patient's emotions. Similarly, nurses felt that the physicians who were engaging in the faculty development were more likely to respond to patients' emotions and be able to handle conflicts in a productive manner. Some faculty members were also inspired to publish about communication topics. Residents also started to embrace patient-centered topics in their career and research plans. For example, one resident started a teach-back log in clinic. Both residents and faculty felt there were less sarcasm and burnout in the institution.

Our method of appreciative inquiry was also spread through the organization. For example, our Performance Improvement Department carried out two organizational debriefs after particular patient "saves" to review both the processes and procedures involved and to recognize the staff who made the "save" happen.

Most important, we heard from our patients. Many commented on our residents being caring and respectful. Also, for the first time, many patients seemed to enjoy teaching rounds. Before implementing our curriculum, many patients commented on how much they disliked "that time when there is a whole convention in my room and I don't have a clue who they all are." Now, they felt that they gained something from rounds: a better understanding about the plan of the day, or what was wrong with them. We would often ask them for feedback on the resident's communication efforts, and they seemed to enjoy that, too.

CONCLUSIONS

Our efforts to implement a comprehensive curriculum have required a lot of work. But the improvements we have seen have made teaching and taking care of patients more fun. To feel the culture changing around us is exhilarating. Both faculty and residents have stronger relationships with each other, and we provide mutual support.

Most rewarding is the change on our patients. Most of us did not understand fully that patients may have trouble perceiving how much we cared. Teaching scripts have helped make the caring explicit, and that has helped *everybody*.

REFERENCES

Barrier, P. A. "Two Words to Improve Physician-Patient Communication: What Else?" *Mayo Clinic Proceedings*, 2003, *78*, 211–214.

Cottingham, A. H., Suchman, A. L., Litzelman, D. K., Frankel, R. M., and others. "Enhancing the Informal Curriculum of a Medical School: a Case Study in Organizational Culture Change." *Journal of General Internal Medicine*, 2008, *23*(6), 715–722.

Fortin, A. H., Dwamena, F. C., Frankel, R. M., and Smith, R. C. *Smith's Patient-Centered Interviewing: An Evidence-Based Method*, 3rd edition. New York: McGraw-Hill, 2012.

Haidet, P., Kelly, P. A. and Chou, C. "Characterizing the Patient-Centeredness of Hidden Curricula in Medical Schools: Development and Validation of a New Measure." *Academic Medicine*, 2005, *80*(1), 44–50.

National Patient Safety Foundation. "Ask Me 3." Accessed Sept. 13, 2012, at www.npsf.org/for-healthcare-professionals/programs/ask-me-3

ADDITIONAL RESOURCES

Some examples for resources we have found useful in teaching scripts include:

Books

Back, A., and Tulsky, J. *Mastering Communication with Seriously Ill Patients*. Cambridge: Cambridge University Press 2009.

Websites

American Academy on Communication in Healthcare webcampus.drexelmed.edu/doccom/user/

A Physician's Practical Guide to Culturally Competent Care cccm.thinkculturalhealth.hhs.gov/

Section on Doctor/Staff Communication at the California Quality Collaborative Website www.Calquality.org/programs/patientexp/Resources

Planetree Physician Grove planetreegrove.com/

5

Activating Patients Through Access to Information

Patrick A. Charmel and Sara Guastello

I was resting in my hospital bed when the doctor came in to tell me about my liver tests. As she shared with me the results, I just nodded. I could tell she was really busy and probably needed to get to the next patient. She did ask me at one point if I had any questions, but I said no. You see, I have a hearing impairment, and I didn't understand most of what she said anyway. I figured I could read the pamphlets she gave me and maybe ask some questions later. But I think you need a medical degree to understand them. It's really frustrating.
—Jorge

INFORMATION YIELDS ACTIVATION

Today, consumers are subject to a perpetual stream of information flowing over the airwaves, online, and through word-of-mouth. Indeed, seemingly limitless data, evidence, and customer reviews are available to guide even the most minor purchases and decisions. Nonetheless, when it comes to health care—a domain where, by any measure, decisions are of the highest consequence—information often continues to be shared on a need-to-know basis, and those judgments on *need* are all too frequently made by health care professionals with limited input from the patient. When the flow of information is decidedly one way, effective partnerships between patients and caregivers are impossible. A central tenet of the Planetree philosophy is the importance of patients and their loved ones having access to a wide range of health and medical information, including real-time access to their medical record and treatment plan. Access to information must be accompanied by support from caregivers to help patients and families navigate through the facts, options, and guidance provided to them.

Hundreds of focus groups conducted by Planetree over the past several years paint a vivid picture of what patients want from their providers. Like Jorge, they want information presented to them in laymen's terms, free from medical jargon. They want their caregivers to be sensitive to their need for information and level of understanding as they discuss their plan of care, attuned to what information is being absorbed and what may bear repeating. They want time for discussion with their caregivers, without feeling rushed. They want their caregivers to take into account their preferences, beliefs, and values. Many want to participate as integral members of their (or their loved one's) health care team, with decisions being made *with* them, not *for* them. Engaging in a dialogue with patients about their health, options available to them, and implications of choices they make related to treatment and lifestyle "activates" them.

DEFINING ACTIVATED PATIENTS: Patients who are able to: (1) self-manage symptoms/problems; (2) engage in activities that maintain functioning and reduce health declines; (3) be involved in treatment and diagnostic choices; (4) collaborate with providers; (5) select providers and provider organizations based on performance or quality; and (6) navigate the health care system. (Hibbard, Stockard, Mahoney, and Tusler, 2004)

Inherent in the definition of activated patients is that they are informed patients. Empowering patients with information shifts the traditional dynamic of the health care relationship wherein professionals are the active providers of information and care, and patients are consigned to the role of passive recipient. Activated patients take the reins of their health care and wellness, asserting their fitting place as a central member of the care team.

PATIENT ACTIVATION IMPROVES HEALTH OUTCOMES

Patient activation not only leads to more meaningful interactions and richer dialogues between patients and caregivers at the point of care. It is also strongly related to a broad range of health-related outcomes. In one study, researchers found that higher levels of activation were associated with lower probability that the patient would have an emergency room visit, be obese, or smoke (Greene and Hibbard, 2012). Mosen and colleagues (2007) found that more highly activated patients were significantly more likely to perform self-management behaviors, use self-management services, and report high medication adherence. In addition, more highly activated patients were more likely to report higher physical and mental functional status scores, as well as higher satisfaction.

These findings are compelling health care providers around the world to implement interventions aimed at facilitating patients' active involvement and engagement in their care as a cornerstone of their strategies to deliver high-quality, high-value care. However, it is important to acknowledge that, for many, recasting clinicians and patients as partners in shared decision making entails a significant shift both in mindset and action. Even individuals who are highly engaged in other aspects of their lives may revert to deferring to their clinicians as being "in charge" when they perceive their health and well-being to be on the line. Research has shown that the fear of being labeled a "difficult" patient—and the associated fear that reprisal from caregivers will jeopardize their care or the care of the loved ones—was a barrier to patients participating more fully in their own health care (Frosch, May, Rendle, Tietbohl, and Elwyn, 2012; Planetree,

Inc. and Picker Inst., 2008). Knowing this, it is incumbent on patient-centered providers and organizations to be proactive about creating an environment of care supportive of patient activation. In this chapter, we will examine a variety of approaches for creating such an environment through the promotion of access to information.

"NOTHING ABOUT ME, WITHOUT ME"

In most health care delivery systems around the world, activating patients and encouraging shared decision making represents a paradigm shift. In a person-centered health care setting, medical degrees and extensive training are no longer the exclusive measures of expertise. A patient's own personal knowledge about her or his body, personal health history, lifestyle, and what is "normal" for them constitutes its own form of expertise. This becomes the basis for partnership, joint goal setting, shared decision making, and reciprocal communication between patients and caregivers. The essence of this approach has been characterized as "nothing about me, without me" (Delbanco and others, 2001) or "no decision about me without me" (Department of Health, 2010).

Shared Decision Making

Shared decision making and patient activation require that traditional provider-centered care models and tools be reoriented to promote a two-way exchange of information. When they are, patients' medical records, once the exclusive domain of health care professionals, are readily shared with the patients and become the basis for important education. Shift report is moved from the nurses' station to the bedside in order to encourage patients and their families to participate in the dialogue. Discharge education begins on admission with a steady dose of both verbal and written education, hands-on training, and assessment of the patients' comprehension of instructions using bidirectional communication tools. Patients are supported in maintaining personal health records. The questions of patients and their family members are welcomed and adequate time is devoted to answering them. Patient decision support tools, such as option grids (www.optiongrid.co.uk), are provided to patients to help them think through treatment possibilities and the personal implications of different decisions (Mulley, Trimble, and Elwyn, 2012).

Diagnosing Patient Preferences

Activating patients to make their health care priorities and preferences known is not only empowering for patients but for clinicians as well, better enabling them to incorporate patient preferences into treatment recommendations (Mulley, Trimble, and Elwyn, 2012). Treatment discussions extend beyond a recounting of options, risks, benefits, and side effects. They are transformed into true exchanges in which patients are supported in expressing their hopes, fears, and what is most important and meaningful to them. Based on this honest and collaborative exchange between patient and clinician, a mutual understanding about the patient's goals and desires is established, which then guides all treatment recommendations and decisions.

From Page to Practice

Interview current or recently discharged patients to explore how well informed they felt during their recent care episodes, and identify what additional information or education would have been useful to them. Questions to pose include:

- Tell me about how you got information about your medical condition and plan of care. What form(s) did this information take? How else would you have liked to have information provided to you?

- Did you feel included in decisions about your treatment? What was done (or not done) to make you feel that way?

- Where do you usually get information about medical concerns?

SHARED MEDICAL RECORDS

In many health care organizations, the medical record is treated as a classified document, shared among providers but shielded from the probing eyes of the patient and family members lest they see something that wasn't meant for them. Organizations may diligently encourage patients and family members to be knowledgeable health care consumers by providing copious patient education materials, facilitating family meetings, and equipping lounge areas with computers preloaded with links to credible health websites. Sharing the medical record during the care experience, however, can face considerable resistance. Providers may express apprehension that patients will not understand or will misinterpret what is in the record and that sharing the record could make an organization susceptible to litigation. Concerns may also arise that reviewing the record could trigger a barrage of questions which will consume caregivers' time, and that such a policy will compromise the privacy of the records.

In a study of three primary care physician practices that provided their patients with an electronic link to their doctors' notes, Delbanco and colleagues (2012) found that opening up doctors' notes to patients resulted in a number of clinically relevant benefits and minimal concerns. Specifically, of patients who opened at least one physician note, more than 77 percent reported feeling more in control of their care and more than 60 percent reported increased medication adherence. Few (under 5 percent) of the doctors reported longer visits or more time addressing patients' questions outside of visits (under 8 percent).

Shared Medical Record Implementation Strategies

Consistent with the "nothing about me, without me" paradigm shift, in patient-centered health care settings, the real-time medical record becomes a basis for discussion and care planning. Patient-centered hospitals, health centers, and clinics recognize that the true owner of the medical record is the patient. Systems are established that not only remove barriers to patients accessing their records, but proactively encourage them to do so. Examples include:

- In-room signage as a visual cue for patients to ask a nurse if they would like to read their record

- Incorporating a reminder about the accessibility of the record during physician rounds to reinforce the message

- Developing formal processes for patients to request to see their records, and setting aside time for a nurse to review the document with them, clarifying confusing terms or unfamiliar acronyms, interpreting test results, and answering questions

- Providing a comments page to capture in writing patients' questions and notes about what they see in the record, as well as to document their progress from their own perspective

Opening the Record Promotes Patient Safety and Satisfaction

In an organization that promotes open communication and partnerships between patients and caregivers, rarely will the contents of the open record be "new" information to a patient. If the record is merely a recap of previously communicated information, why, then, is a shared medical record policy important? Couldn't this same information be shared in other equally effective ways that won't face as much resistance? This line of thinking overlooks some of the added benefits of sharing the medical record.

Knowing they can access their real-time record (even if they opt not to do so) provides patients with an added measure of reassurance that no information is being kept from them. It also helps to cultivate an environment of trust where effective patient-caregiver partnerships—the foundation of patient safety—can thrive. The shared medical record is also an important risk management tool. Numerous hospitals can point to instances when an error was averted because the patient noticed that important information, such as an allergy or a medication order, was either missing or incorrect in their record.

A study of four hospitals that implemented a shared medical record policy suggests that providing inpatients with access to their open records is also a driver of patient satisfaction. Patients who were told they could read their chart rated their hospital more highly than patients who were not informed of the opportunity to do so (Frampton, Horowitz, and Stumpo, 2009).

From Page to Practice

Convene a group of physicians, nurses, risk managers, and others to develop a list of "what if" scenarios that fuel resistance to adopting a shared medical record policy. (For instance, "What if the patient sees in their record that their diagnosis is cancer?" or "What if the record describes the patient as an alcoholic?") As a group, discuss how each of these scenarios would be handled.

Sharing the Electronic Medical Record

Open medical records have long been a hallmark practice of Planetree hospitals. Dating back to the first Planetree hospitals, nurses would sit alongside a patient, thumbing through the pages of the paper chart, discussing the contents contained within. Today, nurses are just as likely to power up a laptop and "click" through the record as the patient scans the computer screen and asks questions. The advent of the electronic medical record (EMR) has created both opportunities and challenges for patient-centered providers committed to sharing the medical record.

The potential of using the chart review to foster open, trusting relationships is lost when caregivers focus more on the technology than the teaching opportunities. On the one hand, for caregivers not yet comfortable or confident with the new tool, connecting and communicating with a patient at the bedside may fall to the wayside as they focus on keystrokes, drop-down menus, and information fields in the EMR. On the other hand, when the EMR is integrated into the care delivery process and involves the patient, it can become a powerful starting point for dialogue. Thoughtful positioning of the computer at the bedside or in the treatment or consultation room enables the patient to see what is being input without sacrificing eye contact between patient and caregiver. A simple re-angling of the screen can engage the patient and family in a discussion about test results or orders. Other settings have worked with their EMR vendor to develop a streamlined summary screen that can be printed and shared with the patient.

From Page to Practice

Laws enacted to preserve the privacy of patients' personal health information are frequently invoked as an argument against a shared medical record policy. Often, however, these laws are misinterpreted. Conduct some research into the laws and regulations to which your organization is subject to ascertain which regulatory barriers to opening the medical record are valid and which are myths.

FIELD EXAMPLE: **SHARING THE MEDICAL RECORD**

Spaarne Hospital, Hoofddorp, The Netherlands

At Spaarne Hospital, patients are encouraged to view their electronic patient records. Though sharing the medical record is required by Dutch law, in many hospitals access remains difficult, with patients having to overcome many hurdles to see their records. In the spirit of Planetree and in alignment with its mission, leaders at Spaarne Hospital wanted to give patients as much information and control as possible over their stay and treatment. Also the hospital recognized that sharing the record was an important component of being completely transparent and being accountable for the care provided and effective communication about that care. To this end, the hospital not only removed customary barriers that kept patients from accessing their records, but also encourages them to review the information in them. Patients identify any errors in or doubts about information contained in the records. The patients' role, though, is not merely to review, validate, and discuss their records; they also have the ability to contribute additional information. By enabling patients to correct outdated information, such as medications or allergies, the shared medical record also contributes to patient safety and patient satisfaction.

FIELD EXAMPLE: **SHARING THE RECORD BEYOND THE HOSPITAL**

Sharp Memorial Hospital, San Diego, California, USA

Sharp Memorial Hospital, a California nonprofit public benefit corporation, is part of Sharp HealthCare, an integrated health care system offering services across the health care continuum. The system includes seven acute and specialty hospitals and two affiliated medical groups. Sharp Memorial Hospital implemented a robust shared medical records program which encourages patients to review their records and contribute personal progress notes. Daily summary sheets from the electronic medical record are printed out for patients who opt into the My Health Record program. Folders, which include progress note sheets, are provided on admission in which the patient can assemble the paperwork provided to them, and have it on hand in an organized format during follow-up appointments. MySharp.com is an extension of the system's commitment to the patient-centered care principle of access to information. The site offers patients secure electronic access to personal health information, even after they have been discharged from the hospital. Patients can log on to the system and view hospital and Emergency Department discharge instructions. They can also access a snapshot of their medical histories, view lab results, and make follow-up appointments.

USING PERSONAL HEALTH RECORDS TO PROMOTE CONTINUITY OF CARE

Personal health records (PHRs) are gaining prominence as a way that patients can store and manage all of their health information from multiple providers and across episodes of care in one secure location. These records are maintained and kept up to date by the patient (or a proxy). The patient also controls with whom they share the information. The development of such portable tools that are associated with the patient rather than a specific health care setting provides an added measure of cohesion and consistency for patients as they address their care needs across points of care and over time.

As an ongoing record of the patient's health history, medical conditions, test results, treatment plans, medication lists, and wellness goals, PHRs have the potential of demystifying the health care experience, which becomes increasingly important for patients managing multiple chronic conditions. And because the owner of the PHR is the patient, it transcends provider silos, equipping patients with a practical tool for aligning the approaches and all their caregivers.

FIELD EXAMPLE: **HARNESSING TECHNOLOGY TO ACTIVATE PATIENTS, PROMOTE ACCESS TO INFORMATION, AND ENHANCE QUALITY OF CARE**

CPH Mental Health, Wijchen/Rosmalen, The Netherlands

To better meet patients' desires for greater choice in their treatment, CPH Mental Health developed an online treatment platform which offers a variety of treatment programs. The platform enables patients to take an active role in managing their care. In addition, online treatment promotes patient independence. Important barriers to care are removed and choice is offered for "blended care," or combinations of face-to-face contact and assistance via Internet or phone. Blended care leads to faster access and more effective and efficient care while maintaining quality. The person seeking help gets support, but also his or her independence is reinforced. With online help the caregiver never takes over the problem, if only because of the physical distance. The patient controls and determines what happens and can independently read health information at their convenience.

REDESIGNING PATIENT EDUCATION

From Page to Practice

Select one patient education publication frequently provided to patients. Read it through the lens of a patient with low health literacy. What changes would you make to it to accommodate the needs of this patient? Consider the terminology used, the length and complexity of the sentences and paragraphs, the formatting of the document, incorporation of visual aids to illustrate key concepts, and use of white space.

Engage patient and family advisers to review the same piece(s). Compare their recommendations to your own.

Patient-centered hospitals implement a range of educational techniques to ensure that patients get the information they need in a manner they will comprehend. Customized education plans combine printed materials, electronic resources, video, and hands-on training to meet each patient's specific needs and learning style.

Using these varying techniques to impart important information is a good start. Techniques for assessing the patient's comprehension of the material conveyed must also be implemented. Asking the patient if he or she has any questions is not sufficient. Patient-centered providers have adopted a number of techniques to more accurately assess individuals' comprehension of the information provided to them. One approach is the teach-back method. After explaining something, such as the plan of care, a new medication, or discharge instructions, caregivers ask the patient to explain it back to them in their own words. Ask Me 3 (National Patient Safety Foundation) is another approach for enhancing patient education which focuses caregivers and patients alike on ensuring a mutual understanding of three fundamental questions: (1) What is my main problem? (2) What do I need to do? and (3) Why is it important for me to do this? If a patient is unable to answer these three critical questions, the caregiver will adjust the teaching approach until comprehension is confirmed.

Neither teach-back nor Ask Me 3 are tests that must be "passed," and it is imperative that patients not feel embarrassed or ashamed if they are unable to answer the questions. Rather, these techniques are employed in the spirit of partnership to ensure that a caregiver's educational style is aligned with the patient's learning style.

Another important strategy for maximizing time spent on patient education is to engage family members. As families continue to shoulder more of the responsibility for caring for their loved ones, it is crucial that accommodations be made to include them in patient education activities as well.

From Page to Practice

With permission from the patient and the health care professional involved, observe a patient education exchange. What went well? What could be improved? How was the patient's comprehension of the material assessed? If applicable, how was family engaged in the education?

FIELD EXAMPLE: **A TEAM APPROACH TO PATIENT EDUCATION**

Hospital Israelita Albert Einstein, São Paulo, Brazil

At Hospital Israelita Albert Einstein, education provided and needed has long been documented by multiple professionals in different sections of the care plan. In the absence of a coordinated education plan, it was common for the same information to be repeated by different professionals or for lack of information to occur due to the assumption that a topic had been previously discussed. This redundancy or inadvertent omission generated discontent among professionals eager to offer the best guidance to the patient. Such was the impetus for the development of a unified patient education record called the Educational Plan. The Educational Plan is initiated within 24 hours of admission and is gradually completed

(Continued)

with the educational needs identified during hospitalization. All professionals involved in care (such as the nurse, dietitian, doctor, physical therapist, speech therapist, and pharmacist) contribute to the document. The identification of the professional in printed script, the professional discipline (doctor, nurse, nutritionist), and registration number and required legislation and must be documented in every step of the plan.

Essentially, the Educational Plan is a centralized location for documenting education that has been provided, additional information needs, and barriers to learning and communication, such as visual (decreased acuity, blindness, use of visual aids), auditory (decreased hearing or deafness, use of hearing aids) and speech deficiencies (aphasia, dysphasia, slurred speech). Caregivers also log the instructional method(s) used, such as demonstration, verbal guidance, delivery of educational materials, as well as the patient's understanding (verbalizes understanding, able to demonstrate, subject needs strengthening). The need for additional resources and treatments available in the community such as products, services, or courses are included. The printed Educational Plan is compulsory in all charts of inpatients, even when the projected necessary education is minimal.

The hospital encourages the involvement of a parent or caregiver in the educational process to monitor and receive instructions during hospitalization and ensure continuity of care after discharge. For patients under eighteen and over sixty-five years of age the hospital requests the appointment of a "guardian." The partner in care is identified in the plan.

Recently included on the Educational Plan form was assessment of "the patient's right to read their medical records" and "the importance of hand hygiene." Given that these key points of education are common to all patients, inclusion of them as items to cover as part of the Educational Plan ensures that this education has been provided and documented accordingly.

The use of the Educational Plan extends beyond patient education. Cultural, religious, psychosocial, and emotional issues are captured so that they can be accommodated by the care team. For instance, religious and cultural beliefs documented in the plan are considered in developing the patient's dietary plan when dietary restrictions may come into play. When emotional barriers are observed, the psychology service is asked to conduct an assessment.

FIELD EXAMPLE: **REDESIGNING DISCHARGE EDUCATION**

Mid-Columbia Medical Center, The Dalles, Oregon, USA

With a focus on reducing avoidable readmissions of patients with congestive heart failure (CHF), Mid-Columbia Medical Center (MCMC) in Oregon set about redesigning its approach to discharge education. The goal of the "reboot" was to improve upon education while patients were still in the hospital in order to prime them to successfully manage their care once they transitioned to their next care setting. In order to maximize teaching, it was essential that any patient with a history of CHF be identified early on in their hospitalization so that education could be provided throughout their hospital stay, ensuring multiple exposures to the information and opportunities for reinforcement of key concepts. As part of the review of patient charts, any physician notes related to heart failure would trigger notification to nursing staff to initiate CHF teaching. From that point on, daily teaching would occur for the duration of the patient's time in the hospital. In addition to this process improvement, the MCMC team made significant revisions to teaching materials. Patients had historically received a half-sheet-size booklet in small type with dense copy and very few pictures or illustrations. This publication was replaced with a new booklet that was larger, included many pictures, less text, and a larger font. Written at a sixth- to eighth-grade reading level, the new booklet clearly conveys diet restrictions, the importance of weighing oneself, and warning signs. It also features places for the patient to record follow-up appointments and medications. Education continues after discharge as well with

(Continued)

an improved process for making discharge phone calls. Yes-or-no questions were replaced with open-ended questions that better enable the nurses making the calls to assess how well patients understood their discharge instructions. For instance, rather than asking, "Are you weighing yourself?" the nurse now asks, "What does it mean if your weight goes up?" and "How often are you weighing yourself?" Though the length of the calls increased from an average of five to ten minutes to closer to twenty to thirty minutes, staff and patients agreed it was time well spent.

FIELD EXAMPLE: **ACCOMMODATING DIFFERENT LEARNING STYLES AND COGNITIVE ABILITIES**

Fatima Zorg, Nieuw Wehl, The Netherlands

Fatima Zorg is a health care organization in the Netherlands specializing in care for people with minor to severe mental disabilities. To support inclusion, the organization has developed systems and tools to help clients have control over their lives and to support them in making their own decisions. Easy access to information, one of Planetree's components, proved to be a challenge for the organization. Because many clients are unable to read, the Fatima Zorg web page and the Fatima Zorg magazine were not suitable communication vehicles. As an alternative, a special website was developed for clients called www.fatimavoorjou.nl (Fatima for You). A special magazine with the same name was developed as well. Both the website and the magazine heavily feature pictograms and photos to support text. The website also has a read-out-loud function for text, and mouse-over audio for the pictograms. On the website, current and future clients can find all kinds of information about the care and living facilities that Fatima Zorg provides, as well as an events calendar and client council news. The magazine is for and by residential clients and contains more informal information, such as who had a change of address. Examples of the Fatima Zorg client magazine can be downloaded from bit.ly/pOJaGP.

CULTIVATING A TEACHING AND LEARNING CULTURE

Access to information is not limited to the shared medical record, family caregiver education, and discharge teaching. Outside these formalized activities, in Planetree settings teaching and learning is woven into the fabric of care delivery. It occurs at the bedside, in family lounges, in on-site consumer health resource libraries, in consultation rooms, and community meeting spaces.

FIELD EXAMPLE: **BEDSIDE SHIFT REPORT**

Waverly Health Center, Waverly, Iowa, USA

Shift report is a vital nursing function that ensures members of the care team are familiar with any changes in patients' status and their plan of care. Transferring the location of this information exchange to the bedside permits the patient and family members to participate in the dialogue, transforming a routine nursing task into a patient-centered opportunity for teaching and learning, connection and partnership. At Waverly Health Center, replacing the traditional taped report with bedside shift report was a natural extension of the staff's efforts to engage patients and establish open, trusting relationships with them. After conducting research into the literature demonstrating the benefits of bedside shift report and outlining implementation strategies, staff developed a plan for each oncoming nurse to meet at the bedside with the nurse whose shift was ending at the start of each shift (with the exception of the 11:00 p.m. shift—this exception was made in order to protect patients' sleep). The nurses share information vital to the patient's recovery and treatment, and together, engage the patient in a dialogue about how he or she is feeling, any concerns, and a review of goals and progress toward them. A review of patient satisfaction data for six months prior to implementation of bedside

(Continued)

shift report compared to six months post-implementation demonstrated improvements in six survey domains: nurses treat you with courtesy/respect; nurses' attitude toward requests; attention to special/personal needs; nurses keep you informed; staff includes you in decisions about your treatment; and staff worked together to care for you. Nurses also reported a positive impact on their work days. With the hospital's previous system of taped report, it could take up to forty minutes into a shift for a nurse to begin caring for patients. With bedside report, staff members start their shifts caring for patients.

Another approach for maximizing teaching and learning is through *patient information rounds*. These are conducted as an adjunct to traditional rounds with a targeted focus on ascertaining and addressing patients' and families' information needs. Health information specialists trained in assessing literacy levels and cognitive ability are able to provide materials that accommodate each individual's needs. A health information specialist takes the time to get to know the patient and his or her story, and uses that information to tailor the information provided. For instance, a determination is made whether resources for family caregivers are in order or whether information on local support groups would be valuable, or perhaps details on a phone app.

The provision of a *consumer health resource library* (whether a brick-and-mortar library, a virtual one, or a combination of the two) conveys an organization's investment in and commitment to the health and wellness of its community, even outside specific episodes of care. Stocked with a variety of health resources—lay books, medical texts, academic journals, consumer-oriented, disease-specific newsletters, websites and Internet references, instructional videos, fitness and nutrition information, resources on complementary therapies, and more—these libraries are open to the public, and support research guided by a health information professional, as well as self-directed research. Given the vast amounts of information available at the click of a mouse, an important service these libraries provide is vetting websites and helping users navigate up-to-date, credible sites to meet their information needs.

COMMUNITY EDUCATION

Emerging reimbursement and policy incentives stress health promotion (not just disease management) as a fundamental role of health care organizations. Providing community access to credible health information is an important component of any organization's health promotion strategy. This community education can take many forms. By enlisting physicians to teach classes on basic anatomy, the pathology of certain diseases, and strategies for disease prevention, *mini med schools* engage community members in learning about their health and well-being outside of specific episodes of care. Similarly, *web-based patient outreach and education* provide avenues for consumers to learn more about health and wellness topics and have questions answered by a reliable source.

FIELD EXAMPLE: **HEALTH ETALK**

Cooper University Hospital, Camden, New Jersey, USA

Part chat room, part live Q&A, Health eTalk is a unique, modern approach to community health education that combines technology, education, and communication to empower individuals from throughout the community to learn more about their health from the comfort and privacy of their home or office. It gives the public an opportunity to ask physicians specific, health-related questions in writing, and receive genuine expert answers in return. A different expert and topic are featured in the Health eTalk program every other week. Questions are invited in the weeks and days leading up to the "live" event. During the "live" thirty-minute event, previously submitted questions and answers are posted, and additional questions

(Continued)

are accepted and answered by a physician expert. An archive of all the Q&As are maintained indefinitely on the hospital's website where they can be accessed after the "live" event. Physicians and topics are scheduled several months in advance. A variety of factors affect the selection of experts and topics, including the expert's interest and schedule, trends and issues in health care, and hospital goals and initiatives. Health eTalk is particularly successful with broad wellness topics (for example, nutrition, parenting) and those that may make patients feel uncomfortable addressing in person (for example, urinary incontinence, sexual health).

Various communication tools are used to promote Health eTalk, including online newsletters, social media, and print advertising. Using a simple, web-based form, personal medical questions related to the topic are submitted to the physician. The physician is given access to the back-end of Health eTalk, where he or she can monitor questions and begin drafting answers. Physicians can work on this at their own pace, from any computer with Internet access.

Health eTalk can be the "gift that keeps giving." For medical staff and other health experts, Health eTalk provides a convenient and low-stress venue for community health education, as well as an opportunity to gain firsthand knowledge on health trends and issues about which patients are truly concerned. Analytics demonstrate that search engines, such as Google and Yahoo!, continue to drive Internet traffic to Health eTalks well after they actually took place. And a "Schedule an Appointment" button on the page of each talk has also resulted in measurable new business for the organization.

CONCLUSION: MEASURING THE IMPACT

Together, the patient education and bidirectional information-sharing strategies described in this chapter foster partnership and communication between clinicians, patients, and their loved ones. These, in turn, promote patient activation and increased *health confidence*, in other words, a patient's confidence in his or her ability to control and manage most health problems or concerns. With the development of patient-centered tools and measures (Coleman, Mahoney, and Parry, 2005; Hibbard, Stockard, Mahoney, and Tusler, 2004), health confidence and patient activation have been converted from "soft" aims into measurable states that can be assessed, quantified, and tied to other outcomes. Indeed, data has demonstrated that improving patients' health confidence can yield significant benefits: improved outcomes, smoother transitions of care, fewer avoidable readmissions, and reduced cost of care (Remmers and others, 2009; Wasson and others, 2006). In fact, a recent study concluded that for those whose overall health is characterized as fair or poor, health confidence is associated with better overall quality of life (Latimer and Lepore, 2012). So, though implementation of these access-to-information strategies may face resistance and may be uncomfortable and perhaps initially time consuming for clinicians, these inconveniences are clearly dwarfed by the potential gains.

REFERENCES

Coleman, E. A., Mahoney, E., and Parry, C. "Assessing the Quality of Preparation for Posthospital Care from the Patient's Perspective: The Care Transitions Measure." *Medical Care*, 2005, *43*(3), 246–255.

Delbanco, T., Berwick, D. M., Boufford, J. I., Edgman-Levitan, S., and others. "Healthcare in a Land Called Peoplepower: Nothing About Me Without Me." *Health Expect*, 2001, *4*(3), 44–50.

Delbanco, T., Walker, J., Bell, S. K., Darer, J. D., and others. "Inviting Patients to Read Their Doctors' Notes: A Quasi-Experimental Study and a Look Ahead." *Annals of Internal Medicine*, 2012, *157*(7), 461–470.

Department of Health. *Equity and Excellence: Liberating the NHS*. London: H.M. Stationery Office. July 12, 2010. Accessed September 19, 2012, at www.dh.gov.uk/en/Publicationsandstatistics/Publications/PublicationsPolicyAndGuidance/DH_117353

Frampton, S. B., Horowitz, S., and Stumpo, B. J. "Open Medical Records." *American Journal of Nursing*, 2009, *109*(8), 59–63.

Frosch, D. L., May, S. G., Rendle, K.A.S., Tietbohl, C., and Elwyn, G. "Authoritarian Physicians and Patients' Fear of Being Labeled 'Difficult' Among Key Obstacles to Shared Decision Making." *Health Affairs*, 2012, *31*(5), 1030–1038.

Greene, J., and Hibbard, J. H. "Why Does Patient Activation Matter? An Examination of the Relationships Between Patient Activation and Health-Related Outcomes." *Journal of General Internal Medicine*, 2012, *27*(5), 520–526.

Hibbard, J. H., Stockard, J., Mahoney, E. R., and Tusler M. "Development of the Patient Activation Measure (PAM): Conceptualizing and Measuring Activation in Patients and Consumers." *Health Services Research*, 2004, *39*, 1005–1026.

Latimer, C. A., and Lepore, M. "Improving the Discharge Transition for the Diabetic Patient." Case Management Society of America Annual Conference, San Francisco, 2012.

Mosen, D. M., Schmittdiel, J., Hibbard, J., Sobel, D., and others. "Is Patient Activation Associated with Outcomes of Care for Adults with Chronic Conditions?" *Journal of Ambulatory Care Management*, 2007, *30*(1), 21–29.

Mulley, A. G., Trimble, C., and Elwyn, G. "Stop the Silent Misdiagnosis: Patients' Preferences Matter." *BMJ*, 2012, *345*, E6572.

National Patient Safety Foundation. "Ask Me 3." Accessed September 2012 at www.npsf.org/for-healthcare-professionals/programs/ask-me-3/

Planetree, Inc., and Picker Institute. *Patient-Centered Care Improvement Guide*. Derby, CT, and Camden, ME: Planetree, Inc., and Picker Institute, 2008.

Remmers, C., Hibbard, J., Mosen, D. M., Wagenfield, M., and others. "Is Patient Activation Associated with Future Health Outcomes and Healthcare Utilization Among Patients with Diabetes?" *Journal of Ambulatory Care Management*, 2009, *32*(4), 1–8.

Wasson, J. H., Ables, T., Johnson, D., Kabcenell, A., and others. "Resource Planning for Patient-Centered Collaborative Care." *Journal of Ambulatory Care Management*, 2006, *29*(3), 207–214.

6

Healing Partnerships: The Role of Family in Patient-Centered Care

Susan B. Frampton, Jeanette Michalak, and
Sara Guastello

*Family is the most important thing in my life. I have two wonderful
daughters and three grandchildren. Nothing puts in perspective the
importance of family like a major health issue. I was diagnosed with
breast cancer last year and was admitted to the hospital for a double
mastectomy. This was my first time spending the night in the hospital
since the birth of my girls over thirty years ago. After the diagnosis,
I was so emotional, so afraid, and I had to do my best to deal with
all the doctors and specialists, to understand the different treatment
options, and keep track of all my appointments. Thank goodness for
my daughters. I relied on them not only for emotional support, but
also to help me ask the right questions and manage all the information
and instructions I was given.*

*My daughters' daily visits to me in the hospital were the highlight
of each day—even though sometimes I slept through the visit. Just
knowing they were there, holding my hand, made being in the hospital a little less scary. My heart would fall when the 8:00 p.m.
overhead page announced that visiting hours were over. One evening
when I was just beside myself with sadness about the road that lay*

ahead, my older daughter pleaded with the nurse so that she could stay a little while longer by my bedside. It made me feel so much better. But the next night, my other daughter's request to stay to a different nurse was rejected. She admonished my daughter that I needed my rest and advised her to come back the next day. My daughter couldn't understand when the rules for visitors applied and when they didn't.

After three days in the hospital, I was discharged. My daughters had already arranged a schedule to stay with me at my house on alternating days to help take care of me during my recuperation. Once I got home, I did my best to tell my oldest the instructions the nurse in the hospital had given me about the dressing changes, since she would be the one changing the bandages that first day home. But I couldn't remember all the details. They told me so many things about my medications, caring for the incision and what warning signs of infection to look out for. Unfortunately, the instructions about the bandages were a blur to me. We just hoped that between the two of us we would figure it out by trial and error.

—Fatima

WHY PARTNERING WITH FAMILY IS GOOD FOR PATIENTS

The epilogue to Fatima's story is encouraging. Her treatment was successful and today, she is healthy and cancer free. Nonetheless, while the ultimate outcome is a good one, Fatima's experience illuminates a multitude of missed opportunities for providing even better care when family is embraced as a vital part of a patient's care team.

In many cultures, hospitals have traditionally relegated family members to the role of visitors. This is not to minimize the profound ways that visitors can lift patients' spirits and bring a healthy dose of companionship, camaraderie, and the comforts of home into the health care setting. Nonetheless, to limit family—those who know the patient best and who comprise their natural support system—to mere *visitation* vastly underestimates the potential for family members to improve patient safety and influence outcomes. Numerous studies have documented that the presence of family minimizes patient anxiety and stress, lowers cardiac complications, and increases patient comfort and satisfaction (see, for example, Fumagalli and others, 2006; Garrouste-Orgeas and others, 2008; Simpson, 1991). This, though, is just the tip of the iceberg when it comes to the capacity of family to have an impact on the patient's health and well-being.

DEFINING FAMILY: In organizations that adopt a patient-centered approach to care, the authority on who is considered family is the patient him- or herself. Family is defined as those the patient considers to be his or her support system.

For some family members, a patient's hospitalization or move to a nursing home provides a welcome respite from the care responsibilities they have assumed. Others may prefer to take on a more active role in caring and advocating for their loved one. For some, the presence of family may *not* be healing. Patient-centered health care organizations support these varying degrees of involvement by first creating avenues for identifying patients' preferences and needs related to the presence of family.

From Page to Practice

Interview current or recently discharged patients to explore the role that their family members play (or played) in their care and treatment. Questions to pose include:

- Tell me about how your family and friends have been/were treated while they were here with you.
- What has been/was done to make them feel welcomed?
- Tell me about any times that your family was restricted from being with you when you would have liked them by your side.
- Describe ways that your family has been/was involved in your care here.

PATIENT-DIRECTED FAMILY PRESENCE

There are few places where the stakes are higher than in hospitals and other health care centers. In hospitals around the world, these high stakes have yielded a multitude of rules and policies intended to standardize processes, minimize risk, and optimize outcomes. Customary among these is the visitation policy which traditionally has established rigid rules about who is permitted to visit patients and when. Such policies frequently impose restrictions on the number and age of visitors, the hours of visitation, and in some cases, the allowable duration of visits. These limitations are well intentioned, but ultimately, unwarranted. More recently, as the patient-centered care movement has gained momentum worldwide, many hospitals have taken steps to liberalize their approach to visitation by minimizing sweeping restrictions to families' presence. In their place, patients, in consultation with their doctors and nurses, determine their own parameters for visitation that will support their personal healing process. Paramount considerations in determining these personal visitation parameters include the patient's preferences and condition and the need to be respectful of the privacy and wishes of other patients in shared rooms.

Beyond minimizing restrictions, adoption of a patient-centered approach to family presence also maximizes the opportunities to engage and educate family members while they are at their loved one's bedside. For instance, the traditional nursing task of shift report (when the nurse whose shift is ending shares information about each patient to the oncoming nurse) can be adapted to a more patient-centered model by involving the patient and family member (with patient consent) in the exchange of information. In addition to relocating the shift report to the bedside, the process can be made more patient-centered by incorporating a discussion of the patient's goals for the day using language understandable by the nonclinicians in the room.

For many hospitals accustomed to restricting visitation during change of shift precisely so this exchange can occur in a timely manner *without* the interference of family members, this adaptation can be met with skepticism. However, one need only consider the time saved later on by having a well-informed, engaged family member serving as a family spokesperson as well as the positive repercussions on the patient's ability to manage his or her care post-discharge to understand the value of inviting family members' presence during shift change.

With the goal of reducing the instances when people are needlessly separated from their support system, many patient-centered hospitals have expanded this liberalized approach to visitation to include allowing family's presence during bedside procedures or even during a code. Support is provided to family members so that they understand what is occurring. Being with the patient can provide comfort for the patient and his or her loved ones, and provide reassurance to family about the care being provided.

TURNING CONCEPTS INTO PRACTICE

The process of adopting a patient-directed approach to family presence can challenge many of a health care organization's most closely guarded conventions. After all, visitation policies not only gained prominence because they ostensibly protect patients' privacy and ability to heal, but also because they are convenient for staff who retain control over when family is and is not present on patient care units. Rounding, shift report, and other important operational practices could be conducted without the intrusion of family overhearing conversations, asking questions, or making special requests. For this reason, it is critical that sites embracing a patient-directed approach to family presence engage staff from a variety of disciplines (including nursing, the medical staff, and security) in developing a policy and nurturing buy-in from the entire organization. (See Table 6.1 for examples of patient-directed family presence policies and guidelines.) The team at Northern Westchester Hospital, a 233-bed hospital in a suburb of New York City and one of the first hospitals worldwide to be recognized as a Planetree Designated Patient-Centered Hospital, implemented patient-directed family presence using the following steps that can be replicated by other organizations (Frampton, 2008):

Step 1: *Educate staff and physicians.* Many studies have been conducted and articles written about the positive effects for both families and clinicians when restrictions on visitation are lifted. Reviewing the evidence-base may be helpful in establishing consensus. Medical Boards and Hospital Infection Control Committees also serve as pivotal committees for discussion, guidance and support.

Step 2: *Identify physician and nursing champions.* These champions serve a vital role as credible subject matter experts and meet with departments to listen and respond to concerns with the ultimate goal of moving the institution toward adoption.

Step 3: *Conduct a pilot study.* Identify a specific area(s) that is willing to pilot patient-directed visitation for a specified period of time. Use the experience of these pilot areas to refine the practice, develop appropriate policies, and educate other departments. Interview patients, families and staff during this period to obtain feedback. Document perceptions and lessons learned for educational purposes.

Step 4: *Establish a time frame for house-wide implementation and finalize visitation policies.* Use the feedback from pilot sites and, whenever possible, have staff from pilot areas accompany champions to new areas to discuss their experiences. Use newsletters, communication boards, etc. to publicize feedback from patients and families about how being with their family, whenever they wanted to, benefitted them.

Step 5: *Publicly recognize your champions for their participation as pilot starters.* Recognition of staff who step out on a limb to support these patient-centered practices is important for acknowledgment and empowerment of staff to embrace and lead other patient-centered initiatives.

Reprinted with permission from the Patient-Centered Care Improvement Guide (www.patient-centeredcare.org)

Table 6.1 Examples of Patient-Directed Family Presence Guidelines and Policies

Hospital	Visiting Guidelines or Policy
Carolinas Medical Center-Mercy, Charlotte, North Carolina, USA	Visitation is valued as an important adjunct to patients' care and comfort. The therapeutic environment, safety of the patient, and personal privacy will be maintained through the approved medical protocols and visitation procedures. Assessment of individual preferences, cultural, spiritual, and special circumstances of patients will be made to provide comfort to patients.
John Hunter Children's Hospital, Newcastle, Australia	Parents/caregivers can visit their child at any time. Parents can sleep beside their child on beds in each inpatient room.
New York Presbyterian/ Westchester Division, New York, USA (Behavioral Health Hospital)	NYP Hospital's policy on visiting hours is generally an open one; that is, 24-hour access to patients for immediate family members. Given the unique clinical nature of psychiatry and the importance of appropriately scheduling multiple daily therapeutic activities for patients (for example, group activities, individual sessions, family meetings, and so on) the Behavioral Health Service Line believes that posting suggested hours facilitates treatment planning and unit programming. The goal is to maximize the benefits patients derive from the array of therapeutic interventions and activities that are offered, and to work collaboratively with patients and their support systems to provide for visitation when there is a need for visits outside posted hours.

(Continued)

Table 6.1   (*Continued*)

Hospital	Visiting Guidelines or Policy
Centre de réadaptation Estrie, Sherbrooke, Quebec, Canada	We acknowledge that the presence and support of your family and loved ones are essential to your rehabilitation. Therefore, we have abolished visiting hours. Your family and friends are always welcome at the URFI. If you so desire we can provide them with a folding bed. We simply ask that you limit the noise level in your bedroom as a sign of respect for other users . . . and that you not forget to attend your therapy sessions.

FIELD EXAMPLE: **BALANCING PATIENT PRIVACY AND FAMILY PRESENCE IN SHARED ROOMS AND WARDS**

Gemini Hospital, Den Helder, The Netherlands

At Gemini Hospital, most patients are admitted to five- to six-bed wards. These physical constraints of the facility were concerning to staff and hospital leadership as they considered the impact of liberalizing visitation on patients in these shared rooms. The hospital's active and influential Client Council, composed of recent patients and family members, also expressed reservations that the unrestricted presence of fellow patients' loved ones could be disconcerting and detrimental to their healing process. Among their concerns was that patients' ability to rest and to eat in privacy would be compromised. Of further concern was that the unrestricted presence of family could undermine staff's ability to provide optimal care if patients refrained from asking personal questions, communicating their needs, or providing intimate details about their physical condition or emotional state within earshot of strangers present to visit fellow patients.

Nonetheless, recognized as a pioneer in patient-centered care in The Netherlands, the hospital was committed to finding ways to liberalize visitation in a way that would be agreeable to patients, family, and staff alike. An essential first step was clarifying the difference between *open* visitation and *patient-directed* visitation in order to debunk the misconception that there would be no controls on visitation. In a patient-directed approach, patients are asked who they need to have with them and what time period(s) it is important to have this person or persons by their side. This enables staff to manage the presence of family members by limiting the number of visitors at any one time without inhibiting patients from having the one or two individuals who are their closest support system nearby. To address the very valid concerns about balancing privacy with the patients' desires for their loved ones' presence, staff was prompted to encourage family members to, when possible, relocate visits with their loved one to one of a number of family spaces on the units. These warm and welcoming spaces are accessible to patients and provide a more private space for families to gather. Nurses now orient patients and families to the availability of these spaces and just ask that they be notified if the patient will be leaving the ward to spend some time with family.

From Page to Practice

Walk through a local hospital or nursing home. Conduct an audit of ways in which the organization explicitly or symbolically invites the presence of family members—or conversely discourages their presence. For instance, are there family lounges? Are they clean and well kept? Is there healthy, nourishing food easily accessible to family twenty-four hours a day? Is there signage or announcements that communicate restrictions to family's presence? In patient rooms, are there comfortable spaces for guests to sit? If they wanted to stay overnight at the bedside of their loved one, what accommodations are available for them? Are there shower facilities available? Document what you find and identify changes that can be made to ensure the physical environment is welcoming of family.

FIELD EXAMPLE: **WHEN CULTURAL EXPECTATIONS COLLIDE WITH PATIENT WISHES**

Tane Hospital, Osaka, Japan

Long before such an approach was classified as "patient-directed visitation," many hospitals in Japan welcomed loved ones to stay with patients, even after hours and overnight. To meet the Planetree Patient-Centered Hospital Designation criteria, the team at Tane Hospital in Osaka contemplated how best to convert this unwritten, customary approach to embracing families' presence into a more formal, openly communicated policy. Of utmost importance was to ensure that efforts to comply with the designation criteria did not compromise the ultimate goal of meeting the needs of patients as they relate to visitors.

Hospital leaders hesitated to formalize this approach to visitation with a public announcement that visiting hours had been eliminated, fearing that such an announcement would create problematic consequences for their patients. To do so would have been to overlook an important cultural component to visitation. Japanese culture obliges patients to receive all visitors. Failure to do so would be considered a social offense, and so for many patients the traditional visiting hours were a welcome way to limit visitors without being disrespectful.

The hospital could not take the risk that patient-directed visitation could easily and inadvertently evolve into unrestricted, open visitation. Such a change would certainly fail to meet patients' needs if patients were put into the culturally uncomfortable position of denying visitors when they didn't feel up to company. The team refining the visitation practices feared that a high-profile announcement about the hospital welcoming visitors at any time would leave patients feeling that they had no control over who visits them and when—which was completely at odds with the intent of liberalized visitation.

This scenario illustrates why there is no one-size-fits-all approach to patient-centered care. There must be room for flexibility to accommodate individual preferences and cultural norms, such as those Tane Hospital faced in reviewing its approach to visitation. The ultimate goal of patient-directed visitation is to support patients' healing through the presence of loved ones. If this goal is undermined through proactive posting of an open visitation policy, as depicted by this example, it is incumbent on patient-centered leaders to formulate an alternate means for meeting this underlying aim. For instance, replacing public signage about visitation with a more personalized approach wherein caregivers communicate directly with each individual patient about their ability to control who visits them enables patients to make their wishes known without risk of offending a family member, colleague, or elder.

From Page to Practice

If you work for a hospital or a residential care center, review your organization's visitation policy. Document any sweeping restrictions to visitation. Based on your experiences, are you aware of any exceptions that have been made to those restrictions? What were the circumstances? How would the current policy be different if the standard approach to visitation was a more flexible one and the exceptions to the standard approach were when restrictions are placed on visitors' presence (for instance, in the case of communicable diseases)? Draft a revised visitation policy from this standpoint.

If you don't work for a hospital or health center, look up the visitation guidelines posted on your local hospital's website. Call your local hospital and inquire about visitation guidelines to see if they match what is posted. If you are visiting the hospital or are a patient, look for signs with visitation restrictions and listen for announcements that visiting hours are over. Document any sweeping restrictions to visitation.

BEYOND FAMILY PRESENCE: EMBRACING FAMILY INVOLVEMENT

Even the most liberal visitation policies miss the mark when family members continue to be regarded as visitors rather than as integral members of the care team. The prevalence of chronic conditions increasingly finds patients' interactions with their team of health care providers a very small percentage of their overall efforts to manage their health. In their day-to-day lives outside of acute care episodes, doctors' appointments and home care visits, many patients rely heavily on their families to manage—and in some cases, to provide—their care.

Patient-centered hospitals value the distinctive expertise that family members possess about their loved one's health, medical history, and capacity to manage their care. This is not mere lip service. Processes and systems are implemented to actively involve family in decision making (to the extent desired by the patient) and to develop a genuinely collaborative relationship between health professionals, patients, and family members based on mutual respect and a common aim: optimizing the patient's health and well-being.

Doing so not only enhances patient and family satisfaction. Fundamental to quality of care is effective care coordination and continuity. Unfortunately, in a fragmented health care system, coordination and continuity can be hard to come by. Family members are positioned to be that vital source of continuity. They often naturally assume the role of advocate and health coach, accompanying the patient to doctors' appointments, ensuring that medications are being taken correctly, and that the patient's medical history is communicated to all care providers. The benefits of engaging these instrumental family members as part of the care team, therefore, extend far beyond a single episode of care. Doing so equips family members with the knowledge they need to effectively advocate for their loved one's needs and preferences, to coach them to manage their patient's care in everyday, life and to manage transition from one setting of care to another.

Shifting from welcoming a family's presence to truly embracing their active involvement can also have some important patient safety implications. For instance, typically family members are taught more complicated medical procedures such as trach care, tube feedings, and ventilator management by visiting nurses. Beginning this preparation in the hospital, with reinforcement in the home, increases the family members' comfort level and competence to carry out these tasks in a controlled environment.

Family members who know a patient intimately are uniquely able to detect gradual or subtle changes in behavior or in their physical state. Hospitals that have implemented family-initiated rapid response teams have found that family members can be an invaluable support to clinicians by alerting them to changes in the patient's condition. This is a formalized mechanism for family members to notify staff when they observe an alarming change. Oftentimes, the hospital will set up a dedicated phone line that family can call from the patient's bedside which will trigger dispatch of a rapid response team.

FIELD EXAMPLE: **DESIGNING SYSTEMS TO OPTIMALLY ENGAGE FAMILY**

Centre de réadaptation Estrie, Sherbrooke, Quebec, Canada

Centre de réadaptation Estrie (CRE) is a rehabilitation hospital dedicated to improving the well-being of clients with motor, hearing, visual, language, or speech impairments. The Centre offers primarily outpatient care, but also includes a twelve-bed inpatient rehabilitation unit. The Centre's care philosophy emphasizes the importance of integrating family into the patient's care. Involving family is not the function of a stand-alone

(Continued)

program; rather, it is embedded into every aspect of the rehab experience. Family members participate in therapy and are trained to use the patient's adaptive equipment, and to modify the home environment to make it more accessible. Clients and families are instrumental in the development of the intervention plan, which is developed based on the client's personal goals, lifestyle, home environment, and rhythms of daily life. Understanding the important role that family plays outside of the Centre in supporting the client's therapies and the rehabilitation process, staff provides personalized training to families on the client's needs, such as how to give injections, manage medications, conduct safe transfers, and so forth. This training includes home visits to the family members as well. Staff spends time with family at the client's home to help them modify the premises to meet the client's needs and to provide family members with the tools they need to be effective, efficient, and confident caregivers. Social work support is provided to family to address the emotional and psychological experience of family caregivers.

FIELD EXAMPLE: **FROM EMBRACING THE ROLE OF FAMILY TO FORMALIZING IT**

Good Samaritan Hospital, Kearney, Nebraska, USA

One formalized approach to engaging family in the healing and recovery process is through the implementation of a Care Partner program. The purpose of the Care Partner program is to enhance the quality and experience of patient care by involving a person who has been selected by the patient to participate in care activities during hospitalization or through the continuum of care. The care partner is much more than a consistent visitor. The partner is a member of the care team and accepts mutually agreed-upon responsibilities for participating in care. These goals may include the physical, psychosocial, or spiritual care and comfort of a patient.

A Care Partner program has been in place at Good Samaritan Hospital (GSH) in Kearney, Nebraska, since 2002. Care partners are trained in routine care functions by unit nurses. The involvement of the care partner is specific to the particular patient's needs and is flexible enough to accommodate the interests and abilities of the individual. Activities that the care partner may participate in include: personal care (such as baths, massage, nail care, shaving), vital signs, simple dressing changes, monitoring intake and output, assistance with walking/wheelchair trips, managing the nonpharmaceutical comfort of patients, therapeutic distractions (such as visiting, reading to, assisting with phone calls, managing visitors), discharge planning, acting as spokesperson to family and friends about the patient's progress, and serving as the physician liaison for questions and updates.

Developing a formal program with supporting tools and standardized guidelines addressed the need for consistency with implementation. A Care Partner program description and materials were developed and distributed. The packet includes a "Care Partners are Welcome" invitation to participate as a partner in care. A program description is included in the packet as well as a listing of potential activities the partner may participate in, an orientation program, and a competency check sheet. The involvement of a care partner in an individual patient's care is visually designated by a heart icon in the patient room and then indicated in writing on the care plan. The care partner wears an identification badge so that all staff can include the partner in the care process. This badge also gives the care partner discounts in the cafeteria and gift shops and identifies them during off-hour visits. The care partner is considered a visitor with regard to hospital policies and liability.

There continues to be increasing emphasis on planning for the continuum of care. For elective admissions, care partners are generally

(Continued)

identified prior to inpatient hospitalization. Care partner education and planning for discharge occurs throughout the stay. The plan for discharge is critical to effective transitions to home, home care, or post-acute stays.

Inclusion of care partners in specialty settings may require program modifications. At the Joint Center, the care partner participates in health activities and care from before hospitalization to home. At the Good Samaritan Hospital's Richard Young Behavioral Health Center, the program was modified on the inpatient psychiatric units to focus on education for the family members and support persons in order to provide a stable and safe environment for continued recovery to occur. The program includes a weekly family night centered around education on crisis planning and how to address emotional and psychological crises. Some mental health first aid concepts are presented as well as information using the Wellness Recovery Action Plan Model. On the youth unit, family games and activities are introduced to assist the families in utilizing their recreational time more effectively as a family. A therapist is present to manage difficult family dynamics that arise. A registered nurse answers questions about medications and works with the care partner on issues of nutrition and medications.

Patients and care partners have universally expressed satisfaction about the partnership. Examples include statements of: patients going home sooner due to the training and confidence of the family member, family feeling like a partner in care, staff comments about reductions in call lights and better patient mental orientation, a professional sense that adverse events (for example, falls, tubes out, delays in care) occur less often when a care partner is present, and improved family responses to behavioral issues. In addition, physicians have reported satisfaction with the program due to a reduced number of calls to the physician by family members.

FIELD EXAMPLE: **INVOLVING FAMILY AS MEMBERS OF THE COMMUNITY**

Judith Leysterhof, Hardinxveld-Giessendam, The Netherlands

At Judith Leysterhof, a small-scale long-term care community for psycho-geriatric residents in The Netherlands, residents' family members are valued members of the residential community. They are invited and encour-aged to participate in community activities and rituals and to remain as active caregivers to the extent mutually desired by the resident and family member. This includes encouraging family members' participation in care planning. Relatives are invited to participate in multidisciplinary discus-sions to develop their loved one's care plan. At Judith Leysterhof, the care plan reflects not only the resident's physical care needs, but also lifestyle and preferences as they evolve over time and the resident's personal goals and aspirations. The involvement of family is essential to capturing who the resident *really* is in order to ensure that care and support provided within Judith Leysterhof is personalized and maximizes each resident's independence, dignity, and lifelong learning and growth. When in-person meetings are not possible for family members, accommodations are made to ensure their ability to meaningfully contribute to the discussion over the phone. A key component of the discussion is for the family and staff to mutually determine what tasks related to the resident's care and support family will be responsible for and which will be within the realm of staff. The discussions are not a one-time occurrence at the time the resident moves in to the community. They occur regularly to ensure that family remains consistently apprised of any changes in the resident's needs and that they have the opportunity to influence the care plan. Communication with family members is hardly limited to these formal care planning meet-ings. The resident's "First Responsible Nurse" is the primary point of contact with the family and reaches out to them to share updates about the resident. A special emphasis is placed on contacting family to share positive progress, for instance, when a resident enjoyed a new activity.

From Page to Practice

Consider where in your organization families are naturally embraced as partners in care (for instance, on pediatric units). Interview staff, patients, and family members in those areas about their experiences. What has been done to help them feel like empowered members of the care team? What more could be done? If the approach to family involvement is informal, draft a formal policy that documents the ways family may be involved and the institutional supports to encourage their involvement. You can download sample family involvement policies at www.patient -centeredcare.org/chapters/chapter7e.pdf.

Explore with your Patient and Family Advisory Council opportunities for expanding and formalizing family involvement opportunities.

SUPPORTING THE NEEDS OF FAMILY

The benefits of involving family as formal members of the care team are numerous. However, it is important to recognize it can take a tremendous emotional and physical toll on family members doing their best to understand their loved one's diagnosis and treatment plan, coordinate their care among multiple physicians, and prepare themselves to manage what comes next. Oftentimes, family members don't want to burden the patient with their own fears and concerns and can be left feeling overwhelmed, with little support for *their* needs. Providing adequate emotional, spiritual, psychological, and even physical support for family members' needs can go a long way toward preparing them to continue serving as an effective support system for their loved one. Examples of types of support that patient-centered hospitals provide include:

- Family rooms where family members can rest and take a moment to themselves in close proximity to—but away from—their loved one's bedside

- Free or discounted meals for family to ensure they are getting the nutrition and nourishment they need

- Visits by a social worker, chaplain, or patient/family advocate to speak to the family members about how *they* are doing

- Specially trained volunteers who are available to provide family members a brief respite from staying at the patient's bedside

- Telephone, computer, and Internet access for family members so they can stay connected while caring for their loved one

- Stress-reducing activities for family members, such as roving chair massages, provision of calming music or aromatherapy, or free access to an on-site fitness center

From Page to Practice

Develop a plan to evaluate the family experience with your organization. Approaches could include facilitating a focus group of family members of recent patients, developing a Family Experience Survey, or incorporating questions about the family experience into an existing patient survey. Dimensions of the care experience to get family feedback on include:

- Opportunities for family involvement in care planning and decision making (to the extent desired by the patient)

- Experiences with visitation

- Educational opportunities for family

- Emotional support available

- Accommodations to support family's comfort

- Family members' understanding of how to report concerns related to care, treatment, service, and patient safety issues

- Supports provided to assist the patient and family to manage transitions to the next care setting

CONCLUSION

Formally and informally, with institutional supports and in the absence of them, patients' loved ones are assuming the roles of advocate, health coach, care partner, family spokesperson, and health system navigator—not to mention informal caregiver. Given this, family members are uniquely suited to help bridge the gap between health care episodes and points of care, making them an integral piece of the patient-centered care value equation. Patient-centered health care organizations put in place systems and supports to maximize family members' ability to be effective in these roles. Central to these efforts is the philosophical shift that must occur within the organization and in the minds of individual health care providers that family is not an adjunct to the care team, but an integral part of it.

REFERENCES

Frampton, S. B., Guastello, S., Brady, C., Hale, M., and others. *Patient-Centered Care Improvement Guide.* Derby, CT, and Camden, ME: Planetree, Inc. and Picker Institute, 2008.

Fumagalli, S., Boncinelli, L., Lo Nostro, A., Valoti, P., and others. "Reduced Cardiocirculatory Complications with Unrestrictive Visiting Policy in an Intensive Care Unit: Results from a Pilot, Randomized Trial." *Circulation*, 2008, *113*(7), 946–952.

Garrouste-Orgeas, M., Philippart, F., Timsit, J. F., Diaw, F., and others. "Perceptions of a 24-Hour Visiting Policy in the Intensive Care Unit." *Critical Care Medicine*, 2008, 36(1), 30–35.

Simpson, T. "Critical Care Patients' Perceptions of Visits." *Heart Lung*, 1991, 20(6), 681–688.

7

Healing Environment: Architecture and Design Conducive to Health

Randall L. Carter and Lisa Platt

When I was hospitalized with a fever of unknown origin, my world was essentially reduced to the bleak and sterile hospital room I stayed in for two weeks. My one window faced an air well and the only furniture—a bed and single chair—had a distinctly institutional feel. The presence of family and visitors, allowed to be by my side during visiting hours, brought me solace and evoked the comforts of home— but accommodations for them were scarce, limited to one metal chair. An orchid gifted to me by my mother-in-law became a symbol of life in that otherwise desolate room. It brought natural beauty into a space populated with intimidating equipment and technology. The orchid became a central focus of my attention, a source of strength and reassurance as I struggled to understand my medical condition, what the future held, and what it would take for me to get better.
—Angie

SETTING THE STAGE FOR PATIENT-CENTERED CARE

Vital to health and well-being, the physical environment is a powerful driver of patient-centered care. Or, as Angie's story illustrates, it can undermine efforts to be more patient-centered. Designing patient rooms to accommodate soft seating and sleepover lounge furniture invites family and loved ones to stay with the patient for extended periods so that they can provide needed social support. Easily accessible family lounges equipped with comfortable seating options and Wi-Fi access promote the involvement of loved ones by ensuring they have dedicated spaces to congregate. Open and decentralized nurses' stations encourage partnerships among caregivers, the patient, and family by increasing staff accessibility and eliminating the physical barrier of traditional work stations. Tidy, nicely furnished staff lounges with natural light and access to food and drink provide hardworking staff a restful and restorative place to spend their break. A reading light by the bedside and a bulletin board or shelf where patients can display personal items is a way to bring some of the soothing comforts of home into an unfamiliar environment. The ability to adjust the temperature, the lights, and the window coverings in their rooms can help patients to maintain a sense of control over their environments during a time when many other aspects of their daily lives may feel out of their control. Private consultation rooms provide a space where patients, family members, and caregivers can discuss sensitive matters without feeling they are on display. Incorporating task lights in patient rooms and eliminating overhead paging creates a more restful environment where patients can get the rest they need to heal.

These examples demonstrate ways that the design of a hospital or long-term care community goes beyond surface-level aesthetics. The design of these healing spaces truly sets the stage for patient-centered care delivery to flourish. What's more, a growing body of literature has demonstrated the connection between the physical environment and patient satisfaction and well-being, pain and stress, and reductions in medical errors, infections and falls (Beauchemin and Hays, 1998; Benedetti and others, 2001; Berry and others, 2004; Chaudhury, Mahmood, and Valente, 2003; Golden and others, 2005; Hendrich, Fay, and Sorrells, 2004; Joseph, 2006; Morrison and others, 2003; Ruga, 1989; Topf and Thompson, 2001; Ulrich and others, 2004; Ulrich, 1991; Ulrich, 1984; Zeisel and others, 2003).

From Page to Practice

Think about places you have been that evoke feelings of comfort, serenity, and well-being. Identify specific design, architectural, and aesthetic elements that created this impression. Consider greenery, artwork, architectural elements, cleanliness, and so on. Conversely, think about places you have been that evoke feelings of anxiety or fear. What design elements contributed to these impressions? Looking at these two lists, how do they relate to health care settings you have been in, whether as a patient, a family member, or an employee?

PLANETREE DESIGN PRINCIPLES

Roslyn Lindheim, a founding board member of Planetree and professor of architecture at the University of California, Berkeley, emphasized that the design of health care settings should (Arneill and Frasca-Beaulieu, 2003):

- Welcome the patient's family and friends
- Value human beings over technology
- Enable patients to fully participate as partners in their care
- Provide flexibility to personalize the care of each patient
- Encourage caregivers to be responsive to patients
- Foster a connection to beauty and nature

Through field examples, in this chapter we will spotlight how health care organizations around the world have applied these design principles.

FIELD EXAMPLE: **MAASZIEKENHUIS PANTEIN, BEUGEN, THE NETHERLANDS**

Figure 7.1 Maasziekenhuis Pantein

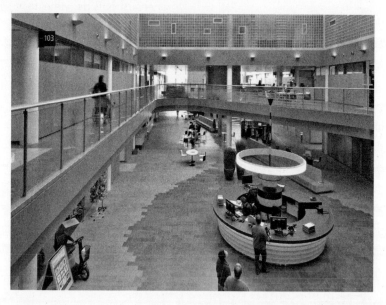

Maasziekenhuis Pantein is a newly built regional hospital which opened in April 2011. Throughout the design process, special attention was given to incorporating Planetree design principles. The building has a tranquil architecture and boasts a welcoming atmosphere and a touch of home.

Featuring a square pond, a garden, and generous footpaths, the setting is inviting. A spacious entrance gives way to a welcoming reception area and a restaurant with an outdoor terrace. Natural light flows throughout the building, even in operating and intensive care rooms. Located just past the reception area, the atrium—an indoor, sunlit court-yard with comfortable chairs and sofas—is a warm space where patients can wait until they enter one of the surrounding outpatient consultation rooms. The pharmacy and a home care shop are also conveniently situated in the atrium. Patient care wards and outpatient consultation rooms are located in different parts of the hospital. The flow for patients and visitors as well as for personnel is separated. This creates peace, clarity, and privacy, especially for the patients.

Private rooms are standard on the wards. All rooms have floor-to-ceiling windows that give patients a generous outside view from their beds. The decor of the room gives the impression of a living room. All rooms have TV and computer facilities with Internet access, offering the patient the opportunity to maximize contact with the outside world and facilitating easy access to information about his illness and other services. The windows and blinds in the rooms can be operated by the patient.

The patient can have a drink or a bite to eat with his visitors or by himself at any given time. By using the computer screen in his or her room, the patient can choose from the extensive menu. In addition, each floor is equipped with its own kitchen and an adjoining lounge.

Family members are welcome to visit their loved ones throughout the day. There are ample accommodations for family members' comfort, such as lounges and cozy corners on the wide corridors. For a loved one wishing to stay overnight with the patient, a chair that folds out into a bed is available.

FIELD EXAMPLE: **HOSPITAL ISRAELITA ALBERT EINSTEIN, SÃO PAULO, BRAZIL**

Hospital Israelita Albert Einstein (HIAE) is considered by América Economía Intelligence as the best hospital in Latin America and was the first hospital in Brazil to be accredited by The Joint Commission International. Its renowned reputation for excellence has been built on its state-of-the-art technology and highly specialized physicians. Today, as the first Planetree Designated Patient-Centered Hospital in South America, HIAE has extended its reputation for excellence to include excellence in patient-centered care.

(Continued)

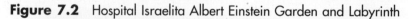

Figure 7.2 Hospital Israelita Albert Einstein Garden and Labyrinth

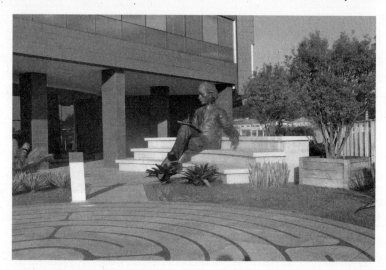

This comprehensive embrace of patient-centered care concepts is reflected in the hospital's physical environment. The design and implementation of the hospital's healing environment was a collaborative process, involving hospital leadership, a team of design experts from Kahn do Brasil Ltda., and, of course, input from customers. The goal was to create a welcoming space and ambiance that would meet the needs of patients, family members, and professional caregivers.

Upon entering, visitors are met with a color palette that resembles sunlight, designed to calm and set minds at ease. Functionality remains of utmost importance, with lighting choices made that not only contribute to a pleasant environment, but most important that support patient safety and facilitate caregivers doing their jobs. Color-coded "zones" within patient rooms create differentiation between family space to one side of the patient bed and staff space where caregivers can easily access the patient room and the decentralized nurse station. With the intention of helping patients feel at home, shelves were incorporated into patient rooms to encourage them to customize their environment with photos, flowers, souvenirs, and accessories. Family caregivers are encouraged to participate in the care and recovery of their loved one. To meet families' needs while they tend to the needs of the patient, rooms are furnished with a comfortable bed and a desk. In addition, each patient floor offers a Family Room appointed with comfortable places to rest, watch TV, eat a snack, make a phone call, or speak with the multidisciplinary team in privacy. Large windows reduce the sensation of being within a closed space, enabling patients to maintain a relationship with the external environment and retain their own circadian rhythms.

Artwork and prints that adorn the walls feature landscapes with a sense of open space to promote healing and restoration. The team specifically selected images featuring trees, nature, birds, butterflies, flowers, and foliage in pairs to avoid being associated with loneliness. A distinctive labyrinth situated next to a statue of Albert Einstein in an outdoor garden area provides a place of peace and solace for patients, family members, and staff. Living areas and convenience services for customers like Cafe Vienna, Drugstore Soares, Safra Bank, and Space Ecumenical all overlook this large healing garden. Convenience services for staff were incorporated in the environment as well. In late 2011, the Reynaldo Andre Brandt Building—Block E opened its doors. The building houses HIAE sectors to support care activities, administration, and logistics. In addition, it features a rooftop employee area including a hairdresser, dentist, banks, a fitness center with external running track, and sites for meditation, massage, and yoga.

FIELD EXAMPLE: **TANE HOSPITAL, OSAKA, JAPAN**

Tane Hospital was established in 1949 as a general hospital and has been responsible for the community health care in the western area of Osaka for more than sixty years. Adjacent to Osaka Dome Stadium (an arena that

(Continued)

Figure 7.3 Tane Hospital Roof Garden

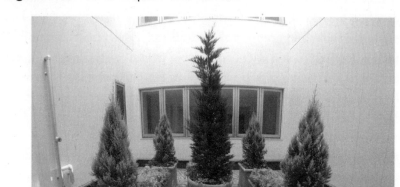

holds 40,000) and the fire department headquarters, the new hospital is located among shopping, restaurants, and other commercial entities of the same joint venture. Accordingly, Tane Hospital aimed to position itself as the urban hospital located at the heart of the currently redeveloping West Osaka district. Further, to function as the lead of the West Osaka district's medical offices in time of disasters, Tane adopted a seismic isolation structure and was designed with an emphasis on functioning smoothly with the fire department (which will be the crisis management control center) and Osaka Dome (which will be the main emergency shelter).

Created with wood-tone material, stained glass decoration, and plants, the entrance and reception area on the first floor is a graceful and welcoming space for patients and visitors. A medical information corner stocked with PCs and books and magazines about health care enables patients and visitors to obtain medical information easily.

The second and third floors house outpatient consultation, physiological function tests, and image diagnosis. Thanks to the large windows on

Figure 7.4 Tane Hospital Interior

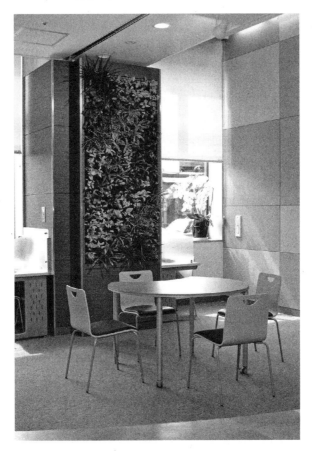

the south side and being on a separate floor and waiting area from the reception area, these floors feature bright and quiet waiting areas.

A restaurant with a view of the pedestrian deck connecting to the surrounding facilities is located on the third floor. The restaurant offers a place of recreation and relaxation for not only the patients and their families but staff as well. These outpatient departments are connected by escalators, so anyone can easily and freely go from one area to another.

(Continued)

The inpatient wards are on floors seven to twelve. Each of the six floors has a different color scheme to minimize confusion for patients, visitors, and staff. Each ward floor was designed with a bright day room with picture windows overlooking the Osaka port. Also, on the seventh floor is a rooftop garden. By improving the inpatient healing environment and enriching the area surrounding their rooms, it was hoped this would encourage the patients to leave their beds and assist in early recovery.

On account of being located in the urban area, Tane Hospital could not be ensured planar spread. Accordingly, departments which required functional connections were vertically placed with dedicated elevators.

On the sixth floor, a day surgery center was installed to provide minimally invasive medical procedures. The Endoscopy Center and OR are on the same floor with the day surgery center to encourage closer cooperation between staffs. As this floor of Tane Hospital is open for business on weekends and holidays, targeting mainly businesspeople, the layout of the sixth floor is designed to be able to complete all medical care and other necessities solely on that floor.

EMPLOYING A PATIENT-CENTERED DESIGN PROCESS

The first day the doors open to a new health center designed with patient-centered principles can be a highly visible way for an organization to demonstrate its commitment to transforming how care is delivered. The behind-the-scenes work, though, that leads up to the public unveiling sets the groundwork for creating a space that meets the needs of patients, families, and staff. First and foremost, a space must be functional. Inviting "end users" (patients, family members, and front-line staff) to share their perspective on what is healing prior to the design development of a space is the only way to ensure that the vision of leadership and the design professionals is aligned with the needs of users. Focus groups, patient experience mapping, patient and staff flow diagramming, listening circles, the creation of mock-up spaces for staff and patients to test out, and inviting leaders, architects, designers and project managers to meet with patient and family advisory councils are just a few of the ways that end users can be engaged in the design process.

FIELD EXAMPLE: **ENGAGING STAFF AND PATIENTS IN THE DESIGN PROCESS**

Elmhurst Memorial Hospital, Elmhurst, Illinois, USA

Figure 7.5   Elmhurst Memorial Hospital Patient Room

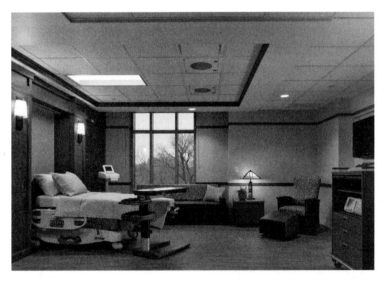

The opening of an 866,000-square-foot, 259-bed replacement hospital in June 2011 was not only an opportunity to replace an outdated building, but also for Elmhurst Memorial Hospital to redefine how it would deliver patient care. The six-year journey that preceded the grand opening began with focus groups with hundreds of staff members, patients, and physicians where participants responded to the questions: *What would your ideal hospital look like? What services would it have?*

(Continued)

These responses became the foundation for the planning of the new hospital. Once initial design concepts were developed, the architects created mock-up patient rooms. More than two hundred patients and 100 percent of staff were invited to view the rooms and share their ideas about what they liked and what could be improved. Patients and staff members tried out different beds before the ultimate selection was made, and the patient bathroom was tested by staff members for several months in order to determine the optimal width of the door and positioning of the toilet, vanity, and shower. Input from the Patient and Family Advisory Council underscored the importance of incorporating white boards into the wall space of patient rooms.

Informed by the feedback of patients, staff, and physicians, the new hospital was designed to enhance healing and well-being. An expansive tree-lined promenade welcomes guests to the campus. Gardens and outdoor seating areas span the front of the building, creating an inviting and nonthreatening first impression. This impression continues upon entering the building. Tall water features and soft overhead music sets a calming tone to the first and second floors. Oversized windows fill public spaces with natural light. Artwork that reflects the local landscape adorns the walls throughout guest and patient areas. All patient rooms are private, including prep, recovery, and treatment areas in the Emergency Department. An on-stage/off-stage concept was incorporated to separate clinical operations from public corridors and spaces in order to maximize patient privacy and efficient workflow. The 90/5 rule ensures that 90 percent of what caregivers need for patient care is available to them within five seconds. Overhead patient lifts were installed in every inpatient room for staff and patient safety.

Welcoming spaces for family were a high priority. Every patient room is divided into three zones: a caregiver zone, a patient zone, and a family zone. The family zone includes two tables and a couch that converts into a bed. Additionally, there are three family lounges and kitchens on each patient floor. The entire campus is Wi-Fi and cell phone friendly. Balconies and atriums are accessible to patients, families, and staff. A retail strip within the hospital features convenience services like a coffee shop and a retail pharmacy. These vendors were selected based on the suggestions of staff and patients. A medical library and resource center open to the community can also be found in this high-traffic area.

Nursing units and outpatient departments are barrier free to accommodate open communication with caregivers and patients. Parking lots are color coded to assist guests in parking adjacent to their destination. Complimentary valet parking is available. Guest services associates greet visitors and assist with wayfinding. Large touch-screen wayfinding kiosks are located at the four main entrances. Green building approaches focused on sustainability as well as impact during construction. Some examples include the use of recycled crushed concrete as the base for sidewalks, installation of 100 percent low-flow plumbing fixtures and lighting occupancy sensors in all nondirect patient care areas. Overall, guided by the patients' and staff members' vision of the ideal hospital, Elmhurst Memorial Hospital was designed to be a welcoming and healing place for its community.

FIELD EXAMPLE: **ENGAGING CLIENTS IN THE DESIGN PROCESS**

Fatima Zorg, Nieuw Wehl, The Netherlands

Fatima Zorg is a health care organization in the Netherlands that specializes in care for people with minor to severe mental disabilities. A guiding principle of the organization is an emphasis on inclusion of clients within their abilities, supporting clients to take control over their lives and in making their own decisions. As a residential institution, the architecture and interior design of Fatima Zorg are the tapestry for the daily lives of clients. Accordingly, the organization set upon devising a process and

(Continued)

tools to engage clients in sharing their impressions and ideas about architecture and interior design. A questionnaire was created using pictograms (easy-to-understand icons) and simple questions. Clients were invited to answer questions about light, smell, sound, landscaping, safety, and signage and were challenged to speak their minds. The findings from the questionnaires are informing future design and construction projects, as well as ongoing renovations and landscaping in existing buildings. For instance, a client answered in the questionnaire that he disliked the smells in the bathroom. An electronic aroma atomizer/nebulizer was installed. Based on client input, trees were planted to create more shaded areas in the garden of a group home and furniture in rooms was rearranged so that clients in wheelchairs could move around more easily. The exercise also brought to light some very simple changes that could be made. A client in a wheelchair answered the question "Do you like the view from your bedroom?" with "I can't really see the view in my bedroom because of the vase with flowers." Supervisors never realized that, as much as he enjoys the flowers, the placement of the vase had the unintended effect of blocking his window view.

WAYFINDING

The incorporation of an integrated wayfinding strategy in the health care environment is essential to optimizing the patient experience. Providing visual cues for wayfinding—signage, landmarks, clear sightlines, and architectural features that include pattern, texture, and color—all can aid in empowering the patient and their loved ones to maneuver through the health care environment independently. However, inclusion of person-to-person assistance in the form of welcome and information personnel also adds an important human component to enhance static building-related orientation indicators.

It is important to acknowledge that the wayfinding process begins as soon as the patient or their companion arrives at the health center campus, so special attention should be paid to building exterior signage, visual markers, and parking direction and orientation. Utilizing "progressive disclosure" (that is, providing information incrementally so individuals can get from one decision point to the next) can assist in guiding patients and visitors in a manner that is logical and does not overwhelm them with too much information all at once.

Consideration of the diversity of patient and visitor demographics is also critical in designing the type and language used for wayfinding. Use of scientific terminology may be confusing to patients. When possible consider substituting more common terms such as "X-Ray" for "Radiology" along with graphic images to improve patients' level of understanding. Also avoid using language and symbols that are distancing, such "NO" and "DO NOT," when not required by code or to ensure patient safety.

From Page to Practice

Enlist community volunteers to serve as wayfinders. Invite them to navigate to specific locations within your campus. Ask them to provide you feedback about their path from the parking lot to their ultimate destination. Use this feedback to evaluate, improve, and augment existing wayfinding devices and systems.

THE AUDITORY ENVIRONMENT

From Page to Practice

Spend a night in a patient room. Share with colleagues what the experience is like. Did you get a good night's rest? Why or why not?

Focus groups with thousands of patients have established sleep and a serene auditory environment as a patient priority (Frampton and others, 2008). Nonetheless, given the beeps and clatter emanating from equipment, the interruptions from overhead pages, and the sound of staff congregating outside of patients' rooms, it is not surprising that in many patient experience surveys, questions related to the auditory environment are among the lowest scoring.

To combat this chronic lack of quiet in today's health care settings, organizations are tackling the issue from multiple fronts. This is vital, as the noises that compromise the healing environment rarely can be attributed to a singular cause. Rounding at night can help to pinpoint the sources of unwelcome noise, such as:

- Loudly closing doors or cabinets
- Squeaky carts and furniture
- High-volume equipment
- Sounds of personnel

Instituting a quiet campaign with highly visible signage and perhaps even a decibel meter to track noise levels can elevate everyone's mindfulness about maintaining a serene auditory environment. A necessary component of any quiet campaign is to provide education to staff, and perhaps even visitors, on the importance of rest for patients.

Beyond efforts to eliminate unwelcome noises, another approach for creating a healing auditory environment is to provide welcome sounds, such as soothing music piped in overhead or channels in patient rooms so patients can choose what they listen to, from healing music to sounds of nature.

The checklist in Table 7.1 is designed to assist organizations in identifying opportunities where changes in the physical environment may contribute to a quieter experience for patients, families, and caregivers.

Table 7.1   Auditory Environment Self-Assessment for Health Care Providers

Single patient rooms	Are your rooms private rooms? Do you still have semiprivate rooms?
Nurse's stations	Are you doing report at a centralized station? Can the nurse stations be reconfigured to smaller areas, with some enclosed rooms? Can you do bedside report? Does the staff have a private, quiet space for meetings?
Finishes in the patient's room	Do you have acoustic ceiling tiles or a hard ceiling? What grade or quality level are they? (Recommend NRC rating of .70 or higher for ceiling tile and .05 or higher for applied floor finishes.)
Finishes in the corridor and other public areas	Do you have acoustic ceiling tiles or a hard ceiling? What grade or quality level are they? (Recommend NRC rating of .90 or higher for ceiling tile and .15–.30 for applied floor finishes) What finishes do you have on the floor (carpet, vinyl composite tile, or sheet vinyl)?
Family consultations	Are these held in the patient's room? If not, do you have a quiet space for family consults to be held?
Carts, equipment, and furniture	Are there squeaky wheels that can be fixed? Replace old and worn wheels with new bearings and silent casters.

(Continued)

Table 7.1 (*Continued*)

Doors and hardware	Adjust door closers and loose hinges, hardware, etc. Install silencers on all doors and cabinets to cushion doors when closing. Consider replacing doors in patient rooms that are below 40 STC for patient rooms and below 50 STC for Mechanical Rooms or rooms with noisy equipment. Check electronic locking systems for silencing or adjustment.
Mechanical systems	Check fan speeds and adjust as necessary. Can silencers be installed on any fans?
Pneumatic tube stations	Are there pneumatic tube stations located near patient rooms? Can you carpet the receptacle, or enclose it within a room?
Patient call systems and paging systems	Can overhead paging be reduced to emergency only? All personal pagers set to vibrate Eliminate walkie-talkies.
Cleaning and maintenance	When does vacuuming and routine floor maintenance typically occur? Could this schedule be modified to limit noisy cleaning practices during hours when patient typically are trying to rest?
Quiet hours	Have you implemented quiet hours, such as times when the lights are dimmed, guests are asked to switch their cell phones to silent/vibrate and keep noise levels to a minimum?
Listening options	Are there multiple options available for patients to choose from for entertainment, distraction, and healing? In semiprivate rooms are there personal devices available that allow each patient to listen to their own choices without disturbing their roommate?

Source: Copyright © Planetree, Inc. Used with permission.

From Page to Practice

Spend a day listening for overhead pages. Count them. How many did you hear in the course of one day? Based on what you heard, how many seemed to be for emergent needs? How many seemed to be more non-emergent reasons? How else could the nonemergent messages be conveyed in a less obtrusive manner?

Spend some extended periods of time in waiting areas during peak patient hours. What are some of the noises you hear? If there is a television, what type of programming is it playing and how loud is the volume? What is the reverberation and echo of sound like in these areas?

Evaluate the auditory environment in check-in and check-out. Do these areas minimize sound transmission for private conversations to take place?

Reducing noise levels is certainly a good place to start for helping patients to get the rest they need and to help reduce anxiety. The restorative potential of sleep will only be optimized, though, when noise reduction strategies are coupled with proactive systems and practices that promote partnerships between patients and caregivers to meet patients' sleep needs. Taking into account patients' sleep patterns when scheduling routine procedures such as blood draws and vital signs is one way of addressing this aim. The Department of Veterans Affairs New Jersey Health Care System uses a sleep assessment tool to ascertain patients' sleep patterns and preferences, as well as to enable the patient to identify nonpharmacological sleep aids (such as sleep masks, sound machines, warmed blankets, and aromatherapy) that he or she may find useful. This sleep assessment opens up a dialogue about why sleep is important and becomes the foundation for supporting more comfortable sleep for patients that will yield the well-documented health benefits of uninterrupted rest.

For those requiring outpatient procedures, having an environment where disruptive and jarring sounds are kept to a minimum will promote an atmosphere that is quiet and soothing and could help in reducing stress.

Using finishes and furniture to help reduce sound reverberation will also enhance the peacefulness of the surroundings as well as improve speech intelligibility. Appropriately designed full- or half-height partitions in check-in and check-out areas can assist in affording visual and auditory privacy to patients.

HEALING DESIGN IS SAFE DESIGN

An aesthetically beautiful health care environment is diminished in value if it is not also functional. Safety is, of course, a chief measure of functionality in any health care building. The interrelation of patient-centered care and patient safety are reinforced by an examination of the healing environment:

- Providing private patient rooms is not only a significant patient satisfier, it also promotes safety by limiting patient transfers, reducing hospital-acquired infections, and supporting more open communication between patients and caregivers. Longitudinal studies and literature reviews indicate significant improvements in ratios of available nurse time for patient care, reduction in medical errors, and reductions in inpatient length of stay (Hendrich and others, 2004; Chaudhury and others, 2003).

- Shifting from centralized to decentralized nurses' stations which keep nursing staff closer to a cluster of patient rooms enables higher levels of observation of patients, which can result in improved assistance and fewer falls (Hendrich and others, 2004). For instance, when The Center for Health Design Pebble Partner Methodist Hospital/Clarian Health Partners in Indianapolis, Indiana, integrated a decentralized nurse station design layout for means of facilitating increased patient observation, measurements of patient falls five years after implementation indicated a 75 percent reduction from previous rates (Center for Health Design Pebble Project Alumni, 2013). This configuration also contributes to noise reduction and reducing interruptions which may lower the risk of medical errors.

- The installation of patient lifts in patient rooms further promotes patient and staff safety. A study of both acute and long-term care health care facilities that had installed patient lifts in rooms indicated a 95 percent reduction in both musculoskeletal injuries and lost days due to injury in clinical staff (Evanoff and others, 2003).

- Ensuring easy access to sinks and hand-washing and sanitizing stations promotes hand hygiene and infection prevention in the most practical of ways. Research indicates that improved compliance in hand hygiene by health care personnel can reduce nosocomial infection rates by as much as 40 percent (Kampf and others, 2009).

- Corridor clutter not only is a safety hazard, making it difficult to maneuver in hallways and to find needed equipment; it can also convey a sense of disorder and inefficiency to patients and loved ones. Creating storage solutions such as centrally located equipment alcoves that keep corridors clear and equipment organized reassures patients that they are in good hands.

Many patients and family members interpret the state of the physical environment of their health center as an indication of overall quality of care. This obliges health care organizations to stay attuned to patients' assessments of the physical environment. Furthermore, a recent study found that hospitals in the highest quartile of performance on patient experience questions related to the environment of care had a lower incidence of selected infections due to medical care (Isaac, Zaslavsky, Cleary, and Landon, 2010).

In an analysis of the root causes of sentinel events in hospitals, communication (or lack thereof) is consistently the most frequent cause at the root of these occurrences. There are numerous design elements that can help to establish connections between patients and caregivers, which support effective partnership and communication, among them:

- Decentralized nursing stations which enable nurses to be more responsive to patients

- Call buttons that emit directly to personal devices held by staff

- Furniture that enables providers to speak to patients at eye level

- Communication boards in patient rooms where caregivers capture the plan for each day, the names of the members of the care team, and patients' goals

- Placement of computer equipment such that caregivers can maintain their personal rapport with patients even as they are inputting information

BALANCING HEALING DESIGN AND SAFETY IN BEHAVIORAL HEALTH SETTINGS

Perhaps nowhere is this delicate balance between patient healing design and safety more apparent than in behavioral health settings. In the interest of protecting patients and staff from harm, the environments of many behavioral health providers have come to more closely resemble prisons than patient-centered hospitals. A number of pioneering patient-centered behavioral health organizations are demonstrating that safety and healing design *can* coexist in behavioral health settings. As just one example, a "soft suicide prevention door" (SSPDoor) has been developed that eliminates many of the hanging hazards associated with a typical door. The door may be easily removed by staff and used as a shield against an attacking patient, and can have calming artwork printed on its face. This door cannot be locked or latched in any manner.

Other ways to incorporate elements of healing health care design without compromising safety include adoption of a well-designed, noninstitutional-feeling color palette, and applying home-like finishes wherever possible to decrease the distance between hospital and home by emphasizing the familiar. Visual access to natural views and daylight provide an empirical link to patients' sense of well-being. Positive distractions such as murals and artwork with calming natural themes also can be a source of stress reduction.

Patients should be able to control their social contact. Design areas enable patients to choose socializing or privacy. Provide enough areas for social gathering so there is not an issue with overcrowding space, and also allow for flexibility in the layout of seating options. Whenever possible, upholstered furniture should be used in both social support and patient rooms to create a comforting atmosphere. Furniture that is heavy and stable and resistant to damage is optimal. Environmental enhancements like these can go a long way toward minimizing the institutional feeling of behavioral health settings, and create an environment that is supportive of healing.

CONCLUSION

The centerpiece of any patient-centered approach to care is the human interaction that occurs between patients, family members, and caregivers. As this chapter illustrates, however, thoughtful design of the spaces where those interactions occur can serve to either promote or undermine those interactions. When compassionate human interactions occur within a space designed to calm, comfort, and heal, the potential for a transformational health care experience can be realized.

REFERENCES

Arneill, B., and Frasca-Beaulieu, K. "Healing Environments: Architecture and Design Conducive to Health." In S. B. Frampton, L. Gilpin, and P. A. Charmel (Eds.), *Putting Patients First: Designing and Practicing Patient-Centered Care*. San Francisco: Jossey-Bass, 2003.

Beauchemin, K. M., and Hays, P. "Dying in the Dark: Sunshine, Gender and Outcomes in Myocardial Infarction." *Journal of the Royal Society of Medicine*, 1998, *91*(7), 352–354.

Benedetti, F., Colombo, C., Barbini, B., Campori, E., and others. "Morning Sunlight Reduces Length of Hospitalizations in Bipolar Depression." *Journal of Affective Disorders*, 2001, *62*(3), 221–223.

Berry, L., Parker, D., Coile, R., Hamilton, D. K., and others. "The Business Case for Better Buildings." *Frontiers in Health Services Management*, 2004, *21*(1), 3– 21.

Center for Health Design Pebble Project Alumni. "Methodist Hospital/Clarian Health Partners." Accessed Apr. 2013 at www.healthdesign.org/pebble/alumni/methodist-hospital/clarian-health-partners

Chaudhury, H., Mahmood, A., and Valente, M. "Pilot Study on Comparative Assessment of Patient Care Issues in Single and Multiple Occupancy Rooms." Unpublished report. Coalition for Health Environments Research, 2003.

Evanoff, B., Wolf, L., Aton, E., Canos, J., and others. "Reduction in Injury Rates in Nursing Personnel Through Introduction of Mechanical Lifts in the Workplace." *American Journal of Industrial Medicine*, 2003, *5*, 451–457.

Frampton, S. B., Guastello, S., Brady, C., Hale, M., and others. *Patient-Centered Care Improvement Guide*. Derby, CT, and Camden, ME: Planetree, Inc. and Picker Institute, 2008.

Golden, R. N., Gaynes, B. N., Ekstrom, R. D., Hamer, R. M., and others. "The Efficacy of Light Therapy in the Treatment of Mood Disorders: A Review and Meta-analysis of the Evidence." *American Journal of Psychiatry*, 2005, *162*(4), 656–662.

Hendrich, A., Fay, J., and Sorrells, A. "Effects of Acuity-Adaptable Rooms on Flow of Patients and Delivery of Care." *American Journal of Critical Care*, 2004, *13*(1), 35–45.

Isaac, T., Zaslavsky, A. M., Cleary, P. D., and Landon, B. E. "The Relationship Between Patients' Perception of Care and Measures of Hospital Quality and Safety." *Health Services Research*, 2010, *45*(4), 1024–1040.

Joseph, A. *The Role of the Physical Environment in Promoting Health, Safety, and Effectiveness in the Healthcare Workplace*. Concord, CA: Center for Health Design, 2006.

Kampf, G., Löffler, H., and Gastmeier, P. "Hand Hygiene for the Prevention of Nosocomial Infections." *Deutsches Ärzteblatt International*, 2009, *106*(40), 649–655.

Morrison, W. E., Haas, E. C., Shaffner, D. H., Garrett, E. S., and others. "Noise, Stress, and Annoyance in a Paediatric Intensive Care Unit." *Critical Care Medicine*, 2003, *31*(1), 113–119.

Ruga, W. "Designing for the Six Senses." *Journal of Health Care Interior Design*, 1989, *1*, 29–34.

Topf, M., and Thompson, S. "Interactive Relationships Between Hospital Patients' Noise-Induced Stress and Other Stress with Sleep." *Heart and Lung*, 2001, *30*(4), 237–243.

Ulrich, R. "View Through a Window May Influence Recovery from Surgery." *Science*, 1984, *224*(4647), 420–421.

Ulrich, R. "Effects of Interior Design on Wellness: Theory and Recent Scientific Research." *Journal of Health Care Interior Design*, 1991, *3*, 97–109.

Ulrich, R. S., Zimring, C., Joseph, A., Quan, X., and others. *The Role of the Physical Environment in the Hospital of the 21st Century: A Once-in-a-Lifetime Opportunity*. Concord, CA: Center for Health Design, 2004.

Zeisel, J., Silverstein, N. M., Hyde, J., Levkoff, S., and others. "Environmental Correlates to Behavioural Outcomes in Alzheimer's Special Care Units." *Gerontologist*, 2003, *43*(5), 697–711.

PART 3

Activating Stakeholders to Create Organizational Change

8

Creating Lasting Organizational Change: Turning Hopes into Reality

Jim van den Beuken and Lucie Dumas

I've been a nursing supervisor for a care center for the past four years and I'm feeling burned out. I became a nurse more than twenty years ago because I felt it was a way that I could make a real difference in peoples' lives. Today, though, my days at work are dominated by documentation, dashboards, budgets, policies, and meetings. There are many evenings when I go home wondering if I made a difference in anyone's life that day. Today, though, I think, will be different, as my organization embarks on an effort to put patient-centered care at the heart of its organizational strategy. Something about this feels different than previous initiatives. I know it will require that we all think differently about how care is delivered, what matters most and my role as a leader. I am excited about what is possible, even though I know it will not be easy, nor will it happen overnight. A spring feeling runs through me. Looking forward to the journey.
—George

BUSINESS AS USUAL IS NO LONGER AN OPTION

Compassionate and devoted health care professionals like George go to work every day motivated by a deep personal conviction to care for their fellow human beings when they need it most. Too often, though, this noble calling is obscured by inefficient health care delivery systems, misaligned financial incentives, rapidly shifting organizational priorities, and other factors that inhibit these professionals from delivering the kind of care they strive to provide. Despite these challenges, most of these caregivers have not lost sight of why they entered the health care profession. They are hungry for change that will enable them to deliver the best possible care to their patients.

At the same time, external pressures from the public, payers, media, policymakers, regulators, and insurance companies are driving health care reform efforts around the world aimed at improving outcomes and reducing costs. Recent research (Klink and others, 2012) indicates that an important cause of unsustainable costs in health care is not aging or unhealthy lifestyles, but the delivery system. Another study indicates that improvements to hospital work and organizational environments may be a relatively low-cost strategy to improve safety and quality in hospitals and to increase patient satisfaction (Aiken and others, 2012).

Suffice it to say, in today's world, change is not an option for health care organizations. It is a requirement. To be sure, this work of transforming culture, humanizing services, and improving the health care delivery system is complex and challenging, but to remain viable, organizations have no choice but to embark on this journey to create lasting organizational change.

BUT HOW?

An organization's capacity for change depends on the readiness, responsiveness, and agility of its employees, leaders, and structures. It involves delivering good solutions today and building capabilities and resilience to respond to future demands. Four principles drive value and can turn hopes into reality:

1. The core: What matters most? What do you hope for?

2. Implementing change to support, nurture, and drive desired performance

3. Connecting knowledge to people: developing, sharing, and adopting exemplary practices

4. Showing meaningful progress: defining, realizing, measuring, and acknowledging excellence

In this section of the field guide, we'll draw on the experiences of the international Planetree network to demonstrate how well-orchestrated organizational change addresses these principles in order to improve the patient experience, create attractive and supportive places to work, and support consistent delivery of high-quality patient-centered care. In addition, we highlight some specific actions organizations can take to turn a vision of change into reality.

FOCUS ON WHAT REALLY MATTERS: WHERE DO WE WANT TO GO?

At its most basic level, excellent care is safe, effective, and compassionate. It is delivered in a healing environment and yields a positive health care experience for patients, family, and caregivers.

This definition of "excellent care" resonates with patients and those who work in health care. Research in The Netherlands ($n = 3,682$) showed that the components of patient-centered care were seen as important both by patients and caregivers. This collective vision for what really matters becomes the basis for a change model that empowers patients and inspires the crucial relationship between caregivers and patients.

Knowing where to go is a good starting point. Knowing where you *are* makes a focused, meaningful pathway possible.

From Page to Practice

As illustrated in Figure 8.1, the Excellerator is a series of steps designed to accelerate improvement by helping you identify your current state, formulate the next steps for reaching your goal, and determine what specifically needs to occur for the change to be realized.

Step 1. Formulate a challenging ambition or hope. What do you hope for?

Step 2. Indicate where you or your project is today using the following scale:

1 = What you hope for is reality. Feedback from others shows it is working. You feel confident in your ability to take action and that what you envision is achieved every day.

2 = You have a plan and feel eager to move forward. You feel motivated to create solutions.

3 = You have several interesting ideas. You feel enthusiastic and interested to explore these possibilities.

Figure 8.1 Excellerator Tool: Creating the Right Movement Ability

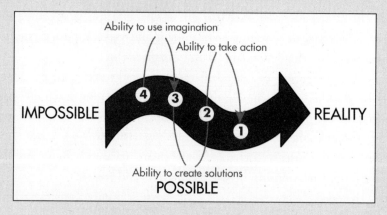

4 = You don't believe the idea is feasible or possible. You feel uncomfortable, stuck or frustrated.

Step 3. Focus on what you or the project needs to move forward.

To move from 4 to 3, focus on the right inspiration

- Envision an attractive future; look for examples.
- Challenge hindering beliefs and emotions.
- Train or develop the ability and power to imagine and build trust.

To move from 3 to 2, focus on the right commitment

- What is your personal commitment to the change? What kind of commitment are you willing to give?
- What do you want/have to invest (time/money)?
- Based on the commitment you are willing to give and the resources at your disposal, is the scope of the project or change appropriate? Does it need to be pared down? Could it be expanded?
- Train or develop the ability and power to solve the right problems and organize the resources needed to succeed.

To move from 2 to 1, focus on the right action

- Identify what to continue, improve, and enjoy.
- Identify what to stop.
- Identify what to start.
- Train or develop ability and courage to take the right action.

Step 4. Act accordingly. Do, listen, learn, and improve until it works.

Source: © Creative Power, www.creativepower.eu; a Next Step app is available for download from www.creativepower.eu

HARNESSING THE POWER OF PEOPLE TO BE THE CHANGE

Transformation starts with individuals who want to change a present situation into something better. Hope and a strong intention are the fire starters. Harnessing this energy to convert it into tangible change involves listening, setting the right climate for initiatives, coping with emotions, and celebrating success. Inform and engage as many caregivers as you can, one at the time. This can be as simple as initiating a dialogue with interesting questions like:

- What would be the ideal care experience and care organization for you?

- What is frustrating you today?

- What are you proud of?

- How would you and your team change?

Though it may seem very basic to begin this work with conversations like these, it is important to note that for many team members, this may be the first time they have been engaged in this kind of honest dialogue about their work and the organization. That, in and of itself, can establish this change effort as different from previous endeavors.

Include or add direct feedback from patients' experiences and outcomes. Often it is quite challenging to bridge individual enthusiasm to collective ambition. It is natural to have many different responses to the change effort in the first phase (see Table 8.1). Questions, ideas, even resistance are indicators that the change effort is starting in a healthy place. If there is no doubt or resistance, the change is probably not well enough understood. A lack of resistance may also be symptomatic of a disengaged or disempowered work force. You can recognize a good start when you hear massive buzz around patient-centered care, spontaneous bottom-up initiatives to improve, and invigorated focus on what really works for patients.

Table 8.1 Responses to Change

Five Constant Facts
1. Early wins help everyone.
2. Honesty keeps you on the moral high ground and able to make the "right" decisions.
3. Early on, people can vacillate between two categories. They will settle into one over time.
4. Personal agendas and personal timelines will dictate an individual's movement from category to category.
5. This is not a one-time judgment. This is a constant fluid continuum that people move throughout.

Five Types of Response to Change		
Who They Are	*Strategies for Engaging*	*Caution*
Champion: Vocal and enthusiastic supporter of the change effort	• Make sure they are heard. Offer a platform to express their opinion. • Make sure they are valid. Inaccuracies in statements can be damaging (sometimes they overpromise due to excitement). • Make sure they want the change that's coming. Ensure that they can conceptualize the vision, not just change for the sake of change.	*Obviously the champion can be your biggest ally, but they can also create the biggest problems. Vet for accuracy and deliberately positive action steps.*

(Continued)

Table 8.1 (*Continued*)

Five Types of Response to Change		
Who They Are	*Strategies for Engaging*	*Caution*
Passive Observer: General population; will follow the masses	• Be patient. Provide frequent and consistent messaging to this group. • This group will respond to passion, but they will need to sustain the change. Provide passionate facts. • Early wins will help move this group. Talking about change can be paralyzing to this demographic so you need to show them.	*Passive Observers will say they want to hear your plan (and they think they do), but the more they hear, the more anxious they will become (whether they agree or not). Get to work early and SHOW them results.*
Silent Spectator: Quiet, without a clear intention of support	• Silence equals silence. It does not equal support or dissent. • Find out why they are silent, and where they are not silent (few people are "always silent"). • Don't wait too long. This is the median group and represents the culture you are trying to change. Leave them dormant for too long and they will create the unwritten aspects of the new culture.	*Assumptions can destroy your efforts with the silent spectator. Learn what is quieting them.*

Table 8.1 (*Continued*)

Five Types of Response to Change

Who They Are	Strategies for Engaging	Caution
Dissenter: loud and vocal opposition	• Listen. Offer them a platform to express their opinion. This opposition group can become your biggest ally. • Make sure they are valid. Inaccuracies in statements can be damaging. (Support their facts). • They hold the key. Regardless of motivations, suggestions or observations from this group can unlock your ability to create the change you desire.	*Determine who they are really. Are they "cantankerous" or "a person with genuine and appropriate concerns" (i.e., committed to the past, troubled by aspects of your approach?)*
Permanent Resister: will not be convinced	• Conserve your energy. No amount of effort will convert them. • Time is vital. Allow enough time to confirm that a staff member is, in fact, a resister (offer positive change, see if it moves them). If unmoved and unwavering, move swiftly to remove them from your future. • Embrace positive attrition. Coach this group onto a more suitable tomorrow.	*Don't make this group your "cause." Separate the dissenters from the permanent resisters (will take a little time) and put your energy toward the dissenters.*

Source: Copyright © Planetree, Inc. Used with permission.

From Page to Practice

As a team, complete the Do Want Matrix to help guide the change effort:

A. What activities and attitudes work well in your team?

B. What new activities and attitudes would you like to see that are not being done today?

C. What existing activities and attitudes do you want to stop?

D. What are lessons learned that can help to guide future efforts?

Source: © Creative Power.

Figure 8.2 Do Want Matrix: Right Action

What are we doing that we don't want? **C**	**A** What are we doing, we want to do
Cease	**Continue**
Waste of health, time, energy, and money. Stop, reduce, or accept.	Perfect, structure, appreciate, sustain.
priority	priority
What are we not doing and we don't want to do **D**	**B** What do we want and are we not (yet) doing
Communicate	**Create**
Lessons learned. Say no, point out who can help or what you can do.	Start and develop. Opportunities and hopes. Creating space. Organize and plan resources.
priority	priority

What Drives Change?

Considering future opportunities or ideals can be hard for people who have to manage many more immediate and pressing problems first. Change is driven by both crisis and opportunity.

- *Crisis* is usually incident driven, such as a mistake, a safety breach, a conflict, or a changed revenue stream. Crisis forces us to change and originates from established routines adopted in the past.

- *Opportunities* are future oriented and define some kind of value or ideal situation that attracts people and resources.

True transformation moves an organization away from this reactionary, crisis-driven approach to change to one that is more proactive with an eye on preventing future crises.

How Can We Help? Create an Enabling Service Climate and Culture

Health care organizations that succeed in transforming the culture to a patient-centered one embed compassion, effective delivery, and high responsiveness into the fabric of everything they do. These organizations have created an "enabling environment" in which certain behaviors are expected, supported, and ingrained in their planning, implementation, reporting, and decision-making systems. Employees feel more vigorous, dedicated, and absorbed in their work. Employee engagement contributes to a service climate and that links to employee performance and customer appreciation and loyalty (Salanova, Agut, and Peiró, 2005; West and Dawson, 2012).

Unfortunately, many health care organizations today operate as "disabling environments." Disabling environments create clutter, confusion, conflicts of interest, and distracting competition for resources. What can be done to initiate the shift from being a disabling environment to an enabling one? Some practical examples include:

- Hiring people who reflect the values of the organization

- Maintaining a pleasant physical environment (cleanliness, noise reduction, clear wayfinding, art, privacy rooms, meeting corners, engaging all the senses)

- Developing professional standards where the expectation of positive and corrective feedback is formalized and practiced

Engaging Caregivers Research demonstrates that engaging professionals drives performance and quality of care. Prins and colleagues (2010) gathered data from a sample of 2,115 Dutch resident physicians and found that doctors who were more engaged were significantly less likely to make mistakes. A study of 8,597 hospital nurses by Laschinger and Leiter (2006) found that higher work engagement was linked to safer patient outcomes.

If you want engaged employees at your workplace (and what leaders don't?), provide jobs that give the opportunity to perform a variety of tasks that employees find meaningful. It is very difficult to be engaged when jobs are experienced as isolated tasks with little connection to the overall mission. An enticing collective mission, motivational goals, and clarity on expectations reduce stress and provide focus for all team members. Caregivers working on what really matters, equipped with sufficient personal and organizational resources, can transform the way health care is delivered.

Organizational resources like training, technology, and systems that promote autonomy remove obstacles at work and have a positive effect on engagement and performance. Thoughtfully developed and targeted training, for example, a patient-centered care retreat, can be helpful for reconnecting employees to their core motivations for working in health care. Experiential curricula emphasize the importance of being present and being courageously engaged in problem solving, sensitize staff to the patient experience, and strengthen competencies around communication and technical skills. It is also important to acknowledge that the medical profession is not a factory, in the sense that if you do A correctly, then B will automatically follow. Professionals encounter a lot of unpredictable situations and outcomes. Acknowledging this helps to build coalitions and participation in improvement initiatives. Ideally all staff members see themselves as caregivers in a multidisciplinary team approach.

Empowering Communication: Interaction, Performance, and Learning

Engagement and communication are closely related. People want to be taken seriously. They want their voices to be heard. This applies in equal measure to both employees and patients, each of whom long for opportunities to share their ideas and concerns, ask questions and contribute to problem solving and decision making.

Patient-centered hospitals make it a priority to obtain regular input from patients and residents, employees, and the community at large. One approach for doing so is through focus groups. This is an example of organizational listening where patients, family, volunteers, doctors, nurses, and support staff are involved and heard. How the findings from the focus groups are shared organization-wide is a critical component to the process. To drive engagement and improvement, focus group findings should be shared broadly, with an emphasis on the following points:

1. How did we understand the feedback from our clients and employees in their own words?

2. What will we keep and what improvements do we make?

3. How is this related to other initiatives (to prevent duplication of work and promote synergy)?

4. What and how are we communicating back to whom?

5. How do we support and monitor progress?

SUPPORT IMPLEMENTATION AND EXECUTION OF EXCELLENCE

While it is important to have a clear vision for where your organization is headed, it is also imperative that the course for reaching that destination be negotiable and adaptable to respond to the continuous adjustment between ambitions, actions, and outcomes. This requires the creation of supportive systems that ensure the change vision remains on course. Important elements of structures that support sustainable change include:

Processes

- Organize all processes around patient behavior and experience.
- Set S.M.A.R.T. (**S**pecific; **M**easureable; **A**ttainable; **R**elevant; **T**ime-bound) goals (Doran, 1981) for team performance and personal development.
- Use *kaizen*, or continuous process improvement methods, for process analyses and improvements.
- Separate ideas from decisions.
- Always involve the people concerned.
- Use one-year and three-year cycles.
- Allow "free" time for ideas to percolate. Not all answers are immediately apparent and not all team members will be most effective in the moment.

Organizational Structure

- Work with results-responsible units.
- Embed client advisory councils in strategic decisions and priority setting.
- Involve employee representatives in strategic decisions.
- Delegate responsibilities as close to the patient as possible.
- Embed meaningful dialogue through focus groups, listening circles, cafés, rounding, walking around, surveys, round tables, and so forth and visibly use this input in improvement efforts and goal setting.
- Appoint a dedicated team member who is able to commit the time required to champion activities related to patient-centered care on an ongoing basis.

- Empower small, self-directed teams to plan and execute their own work.
- Have healing and smart buildings, where people enjoy working and are cued to exhibit patient-centered behaviors, for example, a noise traffic light, privacy rooms, meeting rooms.
- Create IT infrastructure for disseminating and capturing innovative and effective practices.

Methods and Protocol

- Close every day or every week with a seven-minute team evaluation consisting of congratulations, concerns, and one improvement.
- Have patients review protocols and make a patient version of it, such as a patient pathway.
- Expect family to be involved at the intake.

Information and Communication

- Create meetings where hopes, concerns, and complaints are addressed.
- Provide complaint and compliment cards for each other and patients.
- Use open medical records or treatment plans as communication instruments.
- Organize project markets to share progress and motivate people.
- Always multichannel communication, transmitting key messages through personal interactions, accessible documents, and smart processes like text messaging or Yammer.

Decision Making

- Allow small budgets to be allocated on the spot (and require no decision, but accountability).

- Use shared decision making in planning treatment and services.

- Have informal moments for information, inspiration, and support, such as breakfast meetings or luncheon achievement celebrations.

- Shift decision making as close as possible to the patient.

STAYING ON TRACK: DEFINING, MEASURING, AND SHOWING MEANINGFUL PROGRESS

Take time to define what excellence looks like. Choose your measurements before they overwhelm you. Elaborate on what kinds of behaviors, attitudes, service, and outcomes will define patient-centered care for your organization. The challenge is to create supportive systems where progress and coherence is reinforced and makes life as easy as possible. There are many different ways to structure this. You can use measurement to stimulate improvements and morale or to report about achievements. Achievement is a powerful motivator and creates meaning and guidance for future activity. Be sure to include nonmonetary measurements like quality, well-being, or adoption of knowledge.

When patient-centered care is executed well, the vision is broadly embraced, and effective teamwork is practiced daily, then a new type of ambition requires attention: continue to improve, raise the bar, innovate, and increase the impact of good performance to a broader domain or region. Many Planetree affiliates are determined to reach this level. Continue to strengthen the existing basis by providing a nurturing environment for maintaining high performance, hindering complacency, executing tasks well and efficiently, and celebrating successes.

Rarely is the journey to patient-centered care a direct path. It is natural and expected that resistance and reservations may need to be overcome. As the journey progresses, there will be times of great forward momentum, where success builds upon success, and teams support each other in achieving new levels of excellence. Inevitably, though, there will also be times when progress seems to be stalled. Caregivers may become distracted by competing priorities or lulled into a sense of complacency about the patient-centered culture.

These peaks and valleys in the change effort should be anticipated. Finding ways to keep patient-centered care top of mind for all employees, even during periods of change and uncertainty, sets the stage for change that stands the test of time. In order to stay on track, organizations must ensure that employees remain connected to and invested in the change vision, and that all caregivers feel they can contribute to charting the future direction of patient-centered care at the organization. Approaches for doing so include:

- Embedding education on patient-centered care into core competency checks

- Holding "refresher retreats" to reinvigorate the change effort after the initial excitement may have died down

- Promoting dialogue on the current state of the change effort and future directions through articles in organizational newsletters, via the intranet, town hall meetings, and so on

With a strong foundation for patient-centered care in place, organizations can turn their attention to developing new innovative leadership skills, and taking service/business lines to the next level. Research can be initiated or supported to build new scientific evidence on what works.

GUIDING PRINCIPLES FOR THE CHANGE EFFORT

1. *Everyone participates.* Include enthusiastic and critical people and ideas.

2. *Start with yourself.* How would you like to be treated? Believe in what you do and be real.

3. *Listen and be emotionally and intellectually available.* Your patients, families, and coworkers have a need to be heard.

(Continued)

Understanding reduces problems and stress and increases effective problem solving. Put the will to humanize our care, services, and management into action.

4. *State the problem; propose a solution.*

5. *Organize the resources or people necessary to succeed.*

6. *Learn (from the best).* Resistance to learn is denial or a lack of imagination.

7. *Cooperate.* You are not alone. Bundle strength.

8. *Communicate.* Tell why, what, and how. Dare to be a poet and a storyteller. Remember that daily gestures become slowly a need, an expectation, a requirement, and finally a collective commitment.

9. *Enable others to perform better: be kind and competent.*

CONCLUSION: SMALL ENOUGH TO START, BIG ENOUGH TO MATTER

Now is the best moment to do what matters most to patients and caregivers. Make good practices bigger, bad practices smaller, and grow a movement in your organization or your country.

Our work in the health system is so much more than a series of transactions. We have the privilege, in health and social services, to devote ourselves to caring for our fellow human beings. Since one of our values is compassion, our human relations must be a truthful mirror of this. It is a collective work, a shared mission which goes beyond individual (or department) concerns and perspectives.

However, the changes that you make as an individual can have a profound effect on the larger change effort. Small changes can, indeed, matter in a big way. In fact, if you do things differently for thirty minutes every week, you will have changed 50 percent of how you do things in one year. *What thirty minutes will you do differently this week?*

REFERENCES

Aiken, L. H., Sermeus, W., Van den Heede, K., Sloane, D. M., and others. "Patient Safety, Satisfaction, and Quality of Hospital Care: Cross Sectional Surveys of Nurses and Patients in Twelve Countries in Europe and the United States." *BMJ*, 2012, *344*, e1717

Doran, G. T. "There's a S.M.A.R.T. Way to Write Management's Goals and Objectives." *Management Review*, 1981, *70*(11), 35–36.

Klink, A. B., Visser, S., Cools, K., and Kremer, J. *"Kwaliteit als Medicijn: Aanpak voor Betere Zorg en Lagere Kosten."* Booz & Company, 2012. Accessed Apr. 2013 at www.booz.com/global/home/what-we-think/reports-white-papers/article-display/ kwaliteit-medicijn-aanpak-voor-betere

Laschinger, H.K.S., and Leiter, M. P. "The Impact of Nursing Work Environments on Patient Safety Outcomes: The Mediating Role of Burnout/Engagement." *Journal of Nursing Administration*, 2006, *5*, 259–267.

Prins, J. T., Hoekstra-Weebers, J. E., Gazendam-Donofrio, S. M., Dillinghm, G. S., and others. "Burnout and Engagement Among Resident Doctors in the Netherlands: A National Study." *Medical Education*, 2010, *44*(3), 236–247.

Salanova, M., Agut, S., and Peiró, J. M. "Linking Organizational Resources and Work Engagement to Employee Performance and Customer Loyalty: The Mediation of Service Climate." *Journal of Applied Psychology*, 2005, *90*(6), 1217–1727.

West, M. A., and Dawson, J. F. *Employee Engagement and NHS Performance.* Kings Fund, 2012. Accessed Apr. 2013 at www.kingsfund.org.uk/sites/files/kf/employee-engagement-nhs-performance-west-dawson-leadership-review2012-paper.pdf

9

Culture Change and the Employee Experience

Lucie Dumas and Marie-Claude Poulin

At the Centre de réadaptation Estrie, we have a tradition. Once a year, we invite our employees to a general meeting where we offer extensive recognition for their commitment and the quality of their work. This meeting is also a great opportunity to communicate our broad orientations and upcoming projects. The 2004 meeting is still vivid in my mind. It was a time of budgetary restrictions and staff shortages, and we had worked hard to find ways that were both supportive and positive to deliver, once again, the same exacting message: do more and better with less—less money and fewer employees. That general meeting was, however, going to be different. We, the senior management team, had decided our establishment was going to become a Planetree affiliate. We were determined to improve the CRE's strategic positioning with potential employees and with our partners. Having just returned from the Planetree Conference, we firmly believed a new and unexpected path had opened up to brighten our future. It was my turn to speak and I announced to some two hundred employees that within five years the CRE would be ranked

as one of the best employers in Quebec and would become a leader in people-centered health care and management. Nothing less! I had hoped to surprise them, but the surprise was mine. The silence was deafening! Everyone was looking at me. While some people were nodding in approval, there was a good deal of disbelief and polite smiles. I could almost read on their lips: Now what? Is she implying a lack of humanity in the way we treat our patients? A people-centered management style? You really think this is possible when we have to cut positions and increase our workloads? That day, I understood that we had to trace a path between our vision as senior management and their vision as health care workers; that we had to share one ideal; that our culture change would only succeed if every one of us agreed to be a stakeholder in this incredible undertaking.
—Lucie Dumas

SHARED VALUES, BELIEFS, AND VISION

The journey to transform organizational culture to be more patient-centered entails developing the individual and collective commitment of each person involved in actualizing the mission of the organization. Senior management and staff are key actors in achieving this goal, which begins with a clear statement confirming a holistic vision of individuals and their relationship with their environment. From the time an establishment's management team chooses to embark on a culture change journey, its team members promote practices and procedures rooted in daily activities that are coherent with its vision. Knowing how to choose and set priorities is a challenge in coherence, aptly expressed by the motto: "What you do speaks so loudly that I cannot hear what you say!"

To explore the connections between patient-centered care and the employee experience, this chapter will draw on the experience of some twenty member establishments of the Planetree Quebec Network in Canada. Although they have distinctive missions and characteristics, they share common learning experiences that can prove extremely useful to implement patient- and client-centered care and maximize its outcomes. It is often said that winning management strategies require openness to proven models. This is especially true when learning acquired in the working environment is validated by evidence-based data. We will therefore draw on research data collected by the Centre de réadaptation Estrie (CRE), the first Designated Planetree establishment in Quebec (2008), and the architect, in collaboration with the Quebec Ministry of Health and Social Services, of the Planetree Quebec Network (PQN), Planetree International's French-speaking branch.

Devising Tools to Create Meaning

Drawing from Kaplan's strategy maps, Figure 9.1 illustrates how management and staff make choices and perform actions on a daily basis which shape the present and future of their establishments.

The top row establishes the foundations of the organization. The second row positions the organization vis-à-vis its three target clientele groups, the most important being the patients/residents side by side with staff and partners. Employees are considered one of the target groups because their contribution and ongoing support are essential to offer personalized services to the main clientele. This applies equally to partners as services can be enriched through developing community partnerships.

Also situated in the second row are the organization's guiding principles which were adapted from the ten components of the Planetree model (Frampton and Charmel, 2008). The principles act as filters for the decision-making processes described in the third row.

Finally, the fourth row describes benefits or learning (or capital) accomplished by the organization as a result of this decision-making process. Human capital gains take the form of key observable employee attitudes, behaviors, and skills.

Practical Application   This can be illustrated through our concern for attracting and retaining the best employees, which has to be part of the vision at the onset and at the foundational level: *to do our utmost for the wellness*

Figure 9.1 Living in Coherence with Our Foundations

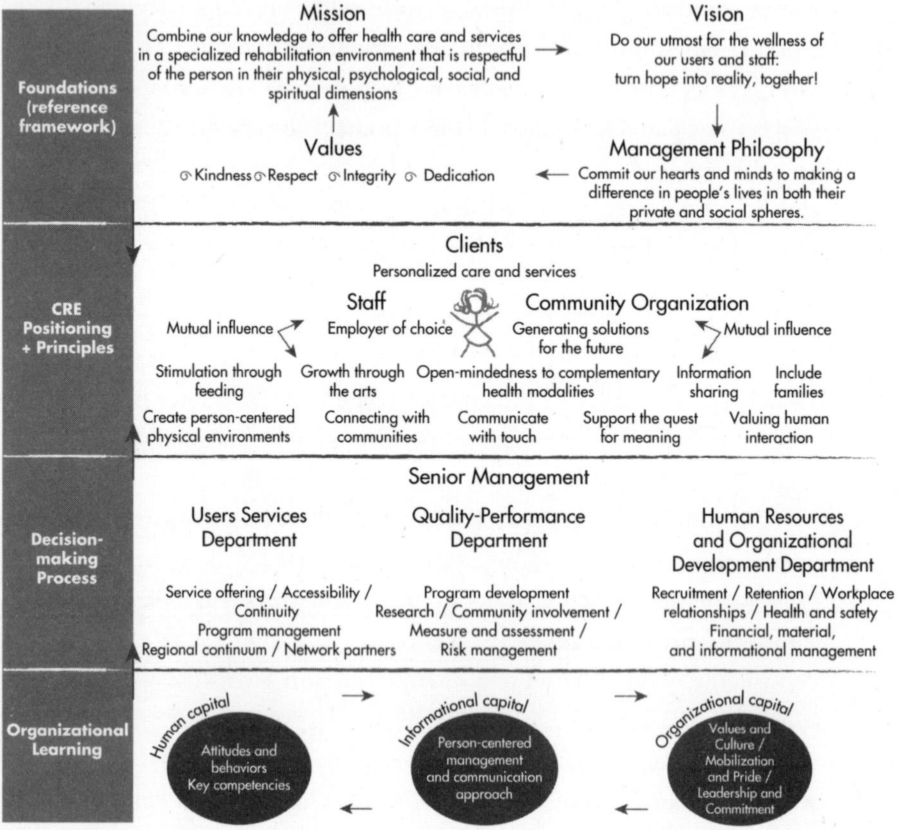

Foundations (reference framework)

Mission
Combine our knowledge to offer health care and services in a specialized rehabilitation environment that is respectful of the person in their physical, psychological, social, and spiritual dimensions

Vision
Do our utmost for the wellness of our users and staff: turn hope into reality, together!

Values
Kindness Respect Integrity Dedication

Management Philosophy
Commit our hearts and minds to making a difference in people's lives in both their private and social spheres.

CRE Positioning + Principles

Clients
Personalized care and services

Staff — **Community Organization**

Mutual influence — Employer of choice — Generating solutions for the future — Mutual influence

Stimulation through feeding — Growth through the arts — Open-mindedness to complementary health modalities — Information sharing — Include families

Create person-centered physical environments — Connecting with communities — Communicate with touch — Support the quest for meaning — Valuing human interaction

Decision-making Process

Senior Management

Users Services Department
Service offering / Accessibility / Continuity
Program management
Regional continuum / Network partners

Quality-Performance Department
Program development
Research / Community involvement /
Measure and assessment /
Risk management

Human Resources and Organizational Development Department
Recruitment / Retention / Workplace relationships / Health and safety
Financial, material, and informational management

Organizational Learning

Human capital
Attitudes and behaviors
Key competencies

Informational capital
Person-centered management and communication approach

Organizational capital
Values and Culture /
Mobilization and Pride /
Leadership and Commitment

Source: Copyright © Réseau Planetree Québec

of our patients/residents and staff. This can be translated into a clear position statement: to be an employer of choice. Chosen strategies and their use must be coherent with the values of patient-centered care. For example, at Centre de rédaptation Estrie (CRE), we strive for transparency in communication to ensure a high quality of human interaction. In addition, we support a structure that promotes empowerment by soliciting the ideas and insights of all stakeholders. For example, we have created a multidisciplinary strategic committee whose mandate is to develop strategies to become an employer of choice.

The decision-making processes are also coherent with patient-centered care values. For example, to ensure high-quality human interaction and promote empowerment, staff members are actively engaged in identifying and prioritizing needs and improvement opportunities. This occurs through surveys and focus groups. Importance is placed on active listening and attentiveness. Assessment results nourish the position, and so on, in an ongoing cycle.

Learning by Experience

The following list of learning opportunities identified in the Quebec experience illustrates our purpose:

1. *To ensure that all members of the senior management team share a common understanding of the basic patient-centered care principles of personalization, humanization, and demystification.* The following questions promote reflection on this topic:

   - To which vision of quality am I ready to commit?

   - Which vision of quality am I ready to communicate?

   - What steps should I follow to help my staff integrate this vision?

2. *To identify the foundations for implementing patient-centered care within the organization,* for example, by noting how the change effort can contribute to the realization of priorities (such as becoming an employer of choice).

3. *To personalize this reflection within each department* (for example, user services, human resources, financial and administrative services, and the like) so as to formulate clear intentions and ensure meaning is created around: (1) our direction through striving for excellence; (2) decisions, including to implement patient-centered care; and, (3) daily activity, where patient-centered principles are used to evaluate the current clinical and management practices in order to improve them and introduce new ones according to need.

From Page to Practice

A vision of quality as being patient-centered promotes a review of job descriptions to ensure that they reflect this organizational commitment of framing delivery and care services around the patient perspective. For example, using this perspective, which proposition best describes the role of maintenance employees: cleaning the workplace or protecting patients from infections? Try this exercise with a few typical employee tasks in your organization.

4. *To integrate the implementation of patient-centered care into the overall organizational improvement plan.* This integration will allow changes to be woven into organizational priorities and strategic positions. As in any process involving change, it is important to adjust the pace according to what the environment will allow. It is also important to assess the actions taken to ensure that they are coherent with the organizational vision in theory and in practice, that they promote the organization and produce the anticipated results.

5. *To consider team meetings as opportunities to reinforce the vision.* This process is time-demanding and must be done gradually, each opportunity bringing a deeper understanding of what it really means and what it takes to be patient-centered. Leadership and staff retreats are optimal places to initiate this process, particularly because participants are invited to reflect on how they wish to bring patient-centered care concepts to life in the organization. It is also important to link the model to components already in place in the organization in order to highlight how changes are related to principles that are now and will always be valued within the organization.

6. *To adopt a systemic approach to communication that takes into account the various steps to transformation in which all stakeholders partici-*

pate. A well-planned communications strategy reinforces existing leadership by clarifying direction and supporting the decision-making process and the evolution of the approach. The plan must take into account the different target groups and ensure convergence of the messages. The messages and the means to convey them will change according to the characteristics and needs of the target groups. Importance should be placed on verbal sharing and feedback in addition to written communication. Particular attention must be given to those entrusted to deliver the messages to ensure they understand the content and feel comfortable delivering and, if needed, justifying the message.

From Page to Practice

To legitimize and guide the organization's decision-making process, it may be to the organization's benefit to develop a specific decision-making tool such as the one developed by the CRDICA (Centre de réadaptation en déficience intellectuelle et troubles envahissants du développement de la région Chaudière-Appalaches). This tool has three distinct steps: (1) assessment of *coherence* of the decision or project, (2) assurance of *collaboration* between all stakeholders, and (3) appraisal of the *relevance* of the decision or project.

Think about a project or decision awaiting action from you. As you map out your next steps, consider the answers to the questions below.

Validating Coherence

- Does my decision or project take into account our organizational values?

- Is my decision or project in line with one of the elements of the organizational vision?

(Continued)

- With which aspects of the strategic plan is my decision in line?
- Does my decision or project take into account the designation criteria of a relevant component of the Planetree model? Which ones?

Validating Collaboration

- Does my decision or project have an impact on other departments? Which ones?
- Has my decision or project been discussed with my team members and other stakeholders? Which ones?
- Does my decision or project require the creation of a project management committee?
- Will my decision or project have an impact on or require the participation of external partners? Which ones?

Validating Relevance

- Does my decision or project bring added value to or improve safety, quality of life, quality of user services; collaboration with family, loved ones, and partners; safety and quality of services offered to staff, the working environment, staff mobilization?
- Will my decision or project generate useful results considering the time and money invested (number of people affected, impacts, duration, costs, influence, innovation . . .)?

QUALITY HUMAN INTERACTION WITHIN A SHARED VISION

The quality of human interaction is the cornerstone of providing patient-centered care, and strongly influences how staff and users value the caregiving environment. Most feel that the people and atmosphere make the greatest difference. Some even say that "it feels good!" How do establishments achieve these results? They aim for ideal attitudes and behaviors and also ask their employees to take part in the process of creating them.

The World Café method (www.theworldcafe.com/) is a particularly helpful tool for this. The CSSS de la Mitis used this method to gather the greatest possible number of ideas from staff on two important questions that concerned everyone: What is not working in my interpersonal relationships at work? What is working? This type of consultation process created a sharing atmosphere—similar to a "café"—that provided real momentum and allowed the organization to gather the essential ingredients to create a charter of attitudes and behaviors for the entire staff to follow.

FIELD EXAMPLE: **DEMONSTRATING THE ORGANIZATIONAL CULTURE FROM THE FIRST DAY AND THROUGHOUT THE ORIENTATION PROCESS**

Centre de réadaptation Estrie, Sherbrooke, Quebec

In patient-centered establishments, the quality of human interaction is manifest from the employee's first day. At the CRE, for example, various procedures for incoming employees have been put in place: a personalized welcome with the head of the program, a "buddy" who helps new employees integrate into the team and familiarizes them with the establishment's layout, and a guided visit highlighting the components of the Planetree model.

As new employees are gradually integrated into the establishment, they discover the required attitudes and behaviors that are valued within the organization. At the CRE, they stem from a reference framework that includes seven indicators:

- Caring for the whole person

- Having respectful attitudes, actions, and behaviors

- Valuing intelligence, judgment, and talent

(Continued)

- Promoting individual commitment
- Recognizing an individual's contributions
- Demonstrating transparency
- Clarifying roles and reciprocal expectations

   Listed in a range of attitudes and behaviors, these indicators constitute the tangible expression of the concepts that define life skills which are considered when staff and managers are evaluated and when managers, staff, and patients are asked to provide periodic organizational assessments.

From Page to Practice

Name a specific attitude or behavior of staff members (employees or managers) that demonstrates each of your organization's values.

FIELD EXAMPLE: **EMPLOYEE RETENTION**

Stamford Hospital, Stamford, Connecticut, USA

At Stamford Hospital, the human resources team developed an employee retention program in 2010 to ensure that employees remain satisfied and motivated and, consequently, maintain a high level of performance. The program requires that managers complete a comprehensive analysis of department-specific retention issues and identify strategies that are unique to their needs. Managers then submit an annual retention plan comprised of initiatives resulting from three main components: the analysis of the real reasons for turnover in the prior twelve months; a risk evaluation of losing high-performing employees; and, finally, the identification of winning retention strategies in the various departments. Within three years of implementing the retention plan, the hospital's turnover has decreased from over 10 to 7.5 percent. First-year turnover decreased even more dramatically, from more than 30 to less than 10 percent. Vacancy rates were reduced from 5.5 percent in 2009 to 2.1 percent in 2012, and a focused effort to fill positions internally resulted in 99 promotions and transfers in 2011, up from 80 in 2009. Finally, in an employee opinion survey, 78 percent of respondents rated the new hire on-boarding process favorably.

The newest component of this retention strategy is an enhanced on-boarding process for new managers to the hospitals. A New Manager On-Boarding Partner orients new managers (whether new to the organization or new to their role as manager), to the organization and their department from a manager viewpoint. The New Manager On-Boarding Partner meets one-on-one with each new manager to review, among other things, the performance management system, reward and recognition systems in place, human resources policies, leadership training available and key contacts for common questions. Each new manager is also connected to another manager in the hospital so that they can begin networking with peers.

Another Success Story

Like Stamford Hospital, the CRE obtained high levels of HR management performance. In the period between 2007 and 2010, the organization's retention rate increased from 94.0 to 98.7 percent. In that same period, the total number of vacant positions was two, though it has remained at zero since 2007. In addition, on its 2009 Quebec Accreditation Council survey, CRE scored a three out of three, the highest rating, on all six dimensions of the survey evaluating employee mobilization. These include fulfillment, involvement, collaboration, support, communication, and leadership. These outcomes have earned the organization a special mention from the Quebec Ministry of Health of Social Services for employee mobilization and valorization.

Recognizing and Supporting Managers' Strategic Position

Managers play a defining role in a culture of wellness in the workplace, as illustrated by the results of a CRE case study on the role of middle management in incorporating the Planetree model within their team (Béliveau, 2011). Their skills in appropriating the model (leading by example), putting the model into practice in their management style, and recognizing these practices among their staff (recognition) influenced the systemic integration of the model. Members of the Planetree Quebec Network jokingly compare the role of middle managers to the cream filling in Oreo cookies. This comparison refers to the managers' strategic position. On the one hand, they must promote and inculcate senior management's vision within their team. On the other hand, they ensure daily care and service delivery by clinical and support professionals.

From Page to Practice

Reflect on your professional experiences. Have you ever witnessed or been told of a situation when a manager had demonstrated a strong presence? Shown recognition? Led by example? If so, what specific actions of this manager come to mind when you think about these leadership activities and qualities? What was the response to it? What were the results?

Daring to Use Person-Centered Approaches and Practices

Over time, a management style based on quality of human interaction also creates an environment conducive to exploring conceptual approaches and practices that highlight human qualities such as commitment, resilience, recognition, or compassion, among others. There also emerges the need to better understand how taking these qualities into account is a powerful tool for continued improvement. To provide indications of the model's efficiency in this area, Marie-Michèle Brodeur and Alexandre J. S. Morin assessed the CRE's organizational health and its average performance over a three-year period in a study conducted from 2007 to 2010. An analysis of the results paints a very positive picture in all clinical and administrative dimensions, which places the establishment in a very good position as an employer. Among the strengths recognized during the three years of data collection are

> the high level of employee commitment toward the organization, their supervisors, colleagues, tasks, profession, and clients (+95%). . . . They [the employees] state that they adopt behaviors coherent with the task description, that improve the ways in which their tasks are effected, and increase the quality of services offered to clients (+95%). . . . Few (3%) intend to leave, resulting in a high level of employee retention. (Brodeur and Morin, 2010)

Organizational Resilience

Aiming to better understand the abilities that contribute to the psychological wellness of its staff, the establishment carried out an initial exploratory study in 2010–2011 on organizational resilience, more specifically on the resilience capacity of the clinical staff on a rehabilitation team. This approach was presented as part of the theme of "Organizational Resilience" at a conference titled *Resilience: New Intervention Perspectives on Rehabilitation* which took place in Montreal in April 2011. Through the use of various scenarios, the clinical staff was invited to look at their own protective factors as individuals and as a group. This was a self-reflective approach, the objectives being awareness, appropriation, and enrichment of these factors. Three strengths emerged from the analysis of this process:

- The team's *capacity to create meaning*, a factor which most likely contributes to maintaining a feeling of coherence in situations of change and instability, this coherence being a gauge of self-confidence

- An evident *sense of humor* within the team and, as a prerequisite, the *ability to step back and see oneself in action,* which helps to view situations of adversity as an opportunity for growth and challenge

- The ability of team members *to stay connected* to one another

After listening to these observations, the clinical staff was invited to put into place ways to support and enrich the identified protective factors. This step in the process (maintenance and development of knowledge acquired over a long period) presented a major challenge because of the many routine daily concerns of the team. The participants met again after six months. Although they admitted that they had not had the time to "deal with" maintaining and enriching these strengths, they recognized that they were always present. It is interesting to note that during this meeting, the newest members of the clinical staff recognized the special nature of this team, a testament to its balance and health.

The overall results from this pilot project lead us to believe that the simple fact of a team becoming aware of its strengths can have positive outcomes for group cohesion. Indeed, the conclusions of research conducted by Jacques Forest, professor and organizational psychologist at the University of Quebec at Montreal, seem to demonstrate that simple awareness of one's strengths has continuous impact over time. Furthermore, we can postulate that, should the team experience adversity, the clinical staff who took part in the project should be able to either call upon existing strengths or replicate the approach on their own (self-empowerment).

Motivation

Reflecting on the theme of the quality of human interaction also invites us to consider the theme of motivation, which requires recognition and a rich architecture of positive behaviors. Mobilization is also a collective effort toward performance. It comes to life in a win-win context and is nourished by human values. We must remember that people tend to commit to causes that confirm their values because they need to give meaning to their actions and relationships, meaning to their lives.

In a study titled *Incentivizing Workers Using Prosocial Motivations*, Ye Li and Margaret Lee (2012) of the Center for Decision Sciences at Columbia University observed that acting for others is a more efficient motivation factor than acting for oneself. After carrying out three experiments to assess whether altruistic behavior is a factor in motivation or not, and if so to what degree, the researchers bring to light the value of the concept of giving back. It is easy to make the connection between this and an organizational culture of patient-centered care where "caring for" is a preferred vehicle for human interaction. For the patients, the experience of care is a positive and reassuring life experience. For the clinical staff, the experience of care is coherent with their deepest aspirations and motivations. For the staff as a whole, whether they are in direct contact with patients or not, activities are person-centered.

Presence and Compassion

Quality human interactions are also based on each employee's ability to be present to the self and to others, and to show compassion. Among others, these qualities are stimulated through staff retreats, which take an experiential format and propose various activities to help employees connect to their deeper motivations, sensitize them to the patient experience, and explore different components of a patient-centered culture. Through this collective experience, which connects employees from all sectors who perform various functions, participants develop a sense of belonging and solidarity that goes beyond their own team to envelop the entire organization. The Planetree Quebec Network has reworked proven programming in American establishments for the Quebec culture which member establishments can adapt and enrich according to their specific needs and mission.

WELLNESS EXPERTS

Beyond standard conventions that all employers must follow to ensure the health and safety of staff, Planetree establishments encourage the promotion of wellness in all its dimensions. This commitment is rooted in the holistic vision of the Planetree patient-centered model. Creativity inherent in interventions is also found in management style, expressed by openness to the expression of talents, to initiative, and to innovation. Each establishment develops, according to its own culture, art therapy or meditation workshops, massage sessions, and new forms of fitness activities, to name but a few examples.

Some establishments have also created committees dedicated to employee recruitment and retention whose role is to keep senior management informed as to the needs and expectations of employees as well as how to ensure that people enjoy their working environment so that they will remain there and attract others. At a time when the balance between work, family, and personal life is a major challenge, employers must be attentive to solutions generated by employees themselves.

CONCLUSION

By valuing intelligence and talent, we mobilize the best in everyone and attract partners that share our aspirations. One employee confided: "Being stimulated in my creativity and having the right to make mistakes is like opening my wings with a safety net under me." Error can be seen as a mistake or as a learning opportunity. In the former, employees prefer to remain in their comfort zone rather than taking risks. In the latter, they venture off the beaten path and become effective channels for promoting innovative ways of seeing and doing. Cultivating its many values and recognizing the person in all dimensions promotes personal fulfillment. In other words, great culture promotes great performance and great competence. This is one of many reasons that explain why so many Planetree establishments stand out at the local, national, and international levels, receiving prizes and awards. For example, since its affiliation with Planetree in 2005, the CRE has been awarded seven prizes and mentions of excellence by the Quebec Ministry of Health and Social Services in the categories of services and management.

A culture such as this stays alive well beyond the people who created it. It is not embodied by one charismatic leader, but by a community of people in constant evolution.

By ensuring the quality and accessibility of care and services, the establishment creates a positive client experience where patients are encouraged to become involved in their own healing process. Quality and accessibility are dependent upon resources, so the establishment will also invest in people-centered management and communication practices through presence, recognition, and leading by example.

The establishment will also be active in the community and, on a larger scale, associate with communities of practice and develop beneficial partnerships because of its reputation. Across the world, Planetree organizations are innovators, ambassadors, and leaders in patient-centered care. In Quebec, they share a common ideal even though their missions are different and they are providing services to very different clienteles. All of them aim to be not only a work environment or a health care environment, but most important, a living environment for staff and patients.

REFERENCES

Béliveau, J. "Le rôle des cadres intermédiaires dans le transfert d'une approche humaniste de gestion, de soins et de services: Une étude multi-cas au Centre de réadaptation Estrie." Doctoral thesis, Université de Sherbrooke, 2011, p. 39.

Brodeur, M.-M., and Morin, A. "Évaluation de la santé organisationnelle du Centre de réadaptation Estrie—Rapport des résultats." Sherbrooke, Sept. 2010.

Frampton, S. B., and Charmel, P. A. (Eds.), *Putting Patients First: Best Practices in Patient-Centered Care.* San Francisco: Jossey-Bass, 2008.

Li, Y., and Lee, M. S. "*Incentivizing Workers Using Prosocial Motivations* (Feb.22, 2012). Available at ssrn.com/abstract=2009873 or dx.doi.org/10.2139/ssrn.2009873

10

Partnering with Patients and Families to Improve Quality and Safety

Edward Kelley, Dennis S. O'Leary, Richard E. Hanke, Susan B. Frampton, Nittita Prasopa-Plaizier, and Anna Lee

On a typical day my wife and I were getting ready for work in the early morning when she suddenly collapsed and went unconscious in front of me. The 911 call and quick response from paramedics got her stabilized and into the emergency room at our local hospital. The cardiologist on duty diagnosed her in need of a pacemaker immediately. The next thirty-five hours following the diagnosis fell into complete disarray. Surgery for the procedure was rescheduled ten times because the surgeon could not be contacted or even found. The hospital staff could give no updates or anticipated plans, and the medical equipment monitoring my wife's vitals failed to work properly. All of this caused me to have my first confrontation with hospital leaders. I demanded to talk with someone in leadership because it was my wife's life they had in their hands. The ultimate outcome was positive, and my wife is doing very well. But those thirty-five hours were full of anxiety and disbelief.

The reaction to my confrontation was one that I did not expect. The chief operating officer, who shortly afterward became president of the health system, showed an extreme desire to use this bad experience as a learning tool for everyone. He asked that I have a conversation with several people in leadership positions. The discussion revolved around what my wife and I had experienced and how we thought it could have gone better. He involved others and when adjustments and corrections were made, they all responded to us with written notes and updates.

A year passed, and I received a call from the president asking if I would like to have a discussion with several other hospital staff and former patients and family members to discuss forming a patient advisory group for the hospital. At the end of that first meeting, I heard a lot about a need for collaboration and the need for listening to patients. I left the meeting wanting to learn more. After three months of listening and questioning, it became apparent that this hospital had a real desire to engage patients and family members in the healing process. The transparency provided a new and invigorating opportunity to view health care in a totally different light. It was a steep learning curve for all of the volunteers wishing to further this "road trip" into the world of health care and the charge of patient-centered care. We had some real supporters in the process because one-third of the newly formed patient partnership council of twenty-eight was staff and leadership at the hospital. The coordinator who listened and supported the whole process for the "outsiders" had a tremendous passion and intuitive knowledge of what could be possible with patient-hospital collaboration in the interest of improving the healing process. The president himself was a champion and let others know within the organization that this advisory group was a good thing for the hospital and not a threat to their work.

The mantra continually used and respected was "Don't decide what should be done with a patient without the patient being directly involved in the conversation." This hospital saw the value of using the patient lens and ultimately had patient representation in the vast majority of continuous improvement processes. The hospital staff became used to stopping conversation to make sure they understood the view-point of the patient. Patient representatives sat at the monthly medical meetings with doctors wishing to promote the true nature of patient-centered care. Patients and family members were on the safety and quality committees.

It is difficult to understand why this collaborative nature of accomplishing such difficult tasks is not commonplace in health care. The value is huge for the consumer and provider. It truly does personalize, humanize, and demystify the fear and potential trauma that comes with serious health concerns. Patient/family advisory groups can become familiar with the complexity of the health care industry, which then allows them to appreciate and celebrate their caregivers. They become true ambassadors to and for the hospital. The hospital can track the data to validate the positive influence on quality and safety results.

The lessons: Find the champion in leadership and a coordinator with a passionate compass. Find people inside and outside the hospital community who want to learn and cause change to occur for the betterment of the health care community; people who are unafraid to ask the question "Why?" and share their energy, insights, and desires to look forward to what ~~can~~ should be.
—Richard E. Hanke, EdD, SPHR

CREATING A CULTURE OF SAFETY AND QUALITY

Nothing focuses the need for a patient-centered care philosophy better than the problem of patient safety. This problem has been prevalent in health care since 400 AD, when Hippocrates first admonished neophyte physicians to "first do no harm." While the attention to patient safety has

---

This section has been adapted in part from an unpublished document entitled "Creation of Cultures of Safety and Quality in America's Health Care Organizations." This document was developed by representatives of The Joint Commission, the Agency for Healthcare

(cont.)

intensified since the 1999 Institute of Medicine report, *To Err Is Human,* recent studies indicate that little or no overall progress has been made in the wake of the report. The net outcome of this improvement shortfall is a continuing stream of avoidable patient harm and deaths.

Where have we failed? There is no dearth of identifiable contributing factors, but the biggest and most obvious shortfall has been the failure to create cultures of safety and quality in health care organizations. Indeed, the *To Err Is Human* report emphasizes that "Health care organizations must develop cultures of safety . . . that are focused on improving the reliability and safety of care for patients" (Institute of Medicine, 1999, p. 14). Among other considerations, such cultures are those that encourage the active participation of patients and their families in improving patient safety.

To some, culture may seem to be a vague concept, but it can basically be defined as the customary beliefs, values, behaviors, and goals that characterize the members of a group (for example, all staff of a hospital, health center, or long-term care community), or more simply "the way we do things around here." The challenge involved in creating positive culture change is embodied in this very definition. Effective culture change literally requires that that the beliefs, values, and behaviors of every single individual in the organization be aligned to make health care quality and patient safety "the" top priority, not simply "a" priority. How does such a culture manifest itself? Here are some important examples:

- Organization leaders—specifically including the CEO and the governing body—are personally invested in quality and safety improvement activities and lead by example. Leaders regularly seek

---

Research and Quality, the ECRI Institute, the Institute for Healthcare Improvement, the Institute for Safe Medication Practices, the Leapfrog Group, the National Patient Safety Foundation, the National Quality Forum, the United States Pharmacopeia, and the Veterans Administration National Center for Patient Safety; however, it has not been formally endorsed by these organizations.

out staff and patient/family concerns and suggestions, act on this input, and share these successes within the organization and publicly.

- The organization provides a positive and secure work environment that enhances staff satisfaction and encourages the retention of staff. Staff members who feel valued and respected are likely to convey similar feelings in the manner in which they care for patients.

- Organization competence in patient care process design and redesign has been established or acquired. Patients and their families are regularly invited to suggest and participate in process improvements.

- The organization encourages and supports the internal reporting of adverse clinical events and near-misses as opportunities for learning and improvement. Patient reporting of such occurrences is encouraged, and mechanisms are created to facilitate this reporting.

- Transparency exists across the organization. When an adverse event occurs, the affected patient/family is given the opportunity to participate in the root cause analysis of the event. Once conclusions from this analysis have been reached, these are shared with the patient/family, and a genuine apology is offered.

- The organization invests the resources necessary to achievement of its health care quality and patient safety goals. This, for example, includes adequate, safe staffing for its patient care services, support for the conduct of root cause analyses, and the proactive identification of patient safety risks.

Consistent with this definition of culture, when a culture of safety and a culture of patient-centered care have been established, they are evident at multiple levels. They are embodied in staff's one-on-one interactions with patients and families at the bedside and in consultations rooms, as well as in organizational governance, strategic planning, and operations.

From Page to Practice

Reflect on the ways that you or, more generally, your organization proactively seek out the opinions and ideas of patients and family members. For instance, are patient focus groups regularly conducted? Do you have a patient and family advisory or patient partnership council? Are patient experience, opinion, or satisfaction surveys administered? If yes, how often? Do patients and family members serve on existing committees or process improvement teams? Is there any patient/family representation on your board of directors? Have you interviewed patients, either during rounds or after discharge, to learn more about their experience? Have you shadowed patients to experience the health care system through their eyes? Have you engaged patients as "mystery shoppers"? What other ways could you engage patients in continuous quality improvement efforts?

The Essential Role of the Patient in Achieving Positive Health Outcomes

There is growing recognition of patients' valuable role as partners in health care (Longtin and others, 2010). Compelled by research demonstrating that engaging patients as essential members of their own health care teams results in greater adherence with their treatment plans and reduces their likelihood of engaging in unhealthy behaviors (Greene and Hibbard, 2012) and that engaging patients and family members can be a viable strategy for reducing avoidable readmissions and follow-up Emergency Department visits (Agency for Healthcare Research and Quality, 2009), many health care providers and policymakers now realize that cooperation from and partnership with informed patients is vital to achieving positive health outcomes.

In late 2010, fifty-eight individuals from eighteen different countries met to consider the role patients can and should play in their health care decisions. The result was the Salzburg Statement on Shared Decision Making, which establishes specific expectations for the roles of clinicians, patients, policymakers, researchers, editors, and journalists in partnering for the delivery of optimal health care (Salzburg Global Seminar, 2010). Among the agreed-upon expectations are

- That clinicians will stimulate a two-way flow of information and encourage patients to ask questions, explain their circumstances, and express their personal preferences
- That clinicians will tailor information to individual patient needs and allow them sufficient time to consider their options
- That patients will speak up about their concerns, questions, and what's important to them
- That patients will seek and use high-quality health information
- That policymakers will adopt policies that encourage shared decision making, including its measurement, as a stimulus for improvement; and
- That clinicians, researchers, editors, journalists, and others will ensure that the information they provide is clear, evidence based, and up to date and that conflicts of interest are declared

A subsequent Salzburg Global Seminar, held in April 2012 with fifty-eight participants from thirty-three countries, built on the themes of the previous meetings with a specific emphasis on reorganizing care delivery to improve population health and drive forward the quality improvement and patient safety agenda in low and middle income countries. The importance of partnership was reinforced in the ensuing call to action that beckoned (Salzburg Global Seminar, 2012):

- Governments to "establish dedicated advocacy and accountability mechanisms and transparent data reporting systems for quality in health care for the population"

- Health policy leaders to "promote interventions that incorporate the use of quality improvement approaches to implement evidence-based, high impact, cost-effective, and client-centered approaches to close the gap between what we know and what we do"

- Communities to "get involved in improving health care at all levels, and actively participate in analyzing information, planning, implementing and evaluating higher quality health care services"

- Health professionals, managers, allied health care workers, and educators to "work towards better health outcomes by meeting evidence-based standards and applying improvement methods to make care more patient- and family-centered as well as culturally appropriate"

- Patients and patient groups to "be involved in the decision-making process of health care delivery, including during their visit to health care facilities" and "develop knowledge and skills to manage their own health problems appropriately, practice healthy behavior and maintain safe living conditions"

The unified voice of this international call for engaging patients and delivering patient-centered care in low- and middle-income countries reflects the critical importance of patient-centeredness in health care across the spectrum of global economic situations.

Engaging Patients in Improving Quality and Safety at the Point of Care

One need only have read the preceding pages of this field guide to be introduced to hallmark patient-centered practices that engage patients and family members at the point of care, and in so doing, set the stage for high-quality, safe care. For instance, *opening up the medical record* as a basis for patient education and conducting *shift report at the bedside* promote an environment of trust and openness in which patients and families understand their voices will be heard and their concerns addressed. Posting the *plan for the day on a communication board* in the patient's room or developing *patient pathways* that document in laymen's terms the typical care and treatment of patients with a specific diagnosis help patients and their loved ones to anticipate what to expect of their care, and importantly, to be able to ask questions or express concerns when the care delivered deviates from what was expected.

This underpinning of transparency is essential for the establishment of effective partnerships between patients and caregivers. When enlisted as true partners, patients and family members can bring up a safety concern or apprehensions about the quality of care being delivered and have it seen as an opportunity—for either (hopefully) averting a safety incident or applying lessons learned so it doesn't happen again.

To encourage patients and family members to report concerns, many patient-centered health centers have developed safety hotlines or campaigns to urge patients to speak up with questions or concerns, or when something just doesn't seem right. The potential difference that one voice speaking up can make is profound. Consider the patient who brings the attention of his doctor to a medication allergy he notices has been omitted from his medical record, averting a potentially dangerous allergic reaction. Or the family member who respectfully asks the nurse whether she has washed her hands prior to caring for his father, limiting the patient's exposure to infection caused by poor hand hygiene. Or the patient who, after falling when trying to reach the toilet on his own after his call light went unanswered, expresses his frustration and humiliation to the staff, reinforcing to them—on a very personal level—the importance of responsiveness.

Another approach for engaging patients and families in quality at the bedside is implementation of patient- and family-activated rapid response teams, which enable those who know the patient best to alert the care team if they notice signs that the patient's condition may be deteriorating.

FIELD EXAMPLE: **TAILORING PATIENT PARTNERSHIP STRATEGIES TO MEET DIVERSE NEEDS**

Centre de Réadaptation en Déficience Intellectuelle et en Troubles Envahissants du Développement de Chaudière-Appalaches (CRDITEDA), Lévis, Quebec, Canada

People who have an intellectual impairment (II) or a pervasive developmental disorder (PDD) often have difficulty both expressing themselves and understanding others. These challenges, though, do not preclude them from being partners in their care and treatment. These patients have important things to say and ideas to contribute, though they may have limited ways to express them. To ensure that their clients are given a voice and are thoughtfully engaged as members of their care team, CRDITEDA has developed a number of strategies for engaging this patient population. To develop these strategies, CRDITEDA went directly to the clients themselves. Two hundred and thirty-four people with II or PDD were interviewed as part of forum to explore what works best for them relative to participating in their care. Among them, fifty-two were elected to represent the whole group during the forum. Based on their input, written documents were developed to meet their needs. Simple language, pictograms, visual cues, and symbols were incorporated to create clear and effective messages understandable by the largest number. Topics focused on areas of greatest interest to the clientele, including the living environment, hobbies, learning and education, and social environment. Even the procedures for electing the delegates were changed from a traditional form of voting to an approach in full color. Each person wishing to be elected as a delegate was associated with a different-colored box. Voters chose the token corresponding to the color of the box associated with the person. The findings from this consultative work were distilled into a unique publicly available, step-by-step guide that establishes a detailed set of standard practices for all organizations wishing to give a voice to their clientele suffering from verbal communication difficulties.

Engaging Patients in Improving Quality and Safety at the Organizational Level

As captured in Richard Hanke's story at the beginning of this chapter, despite our best efforts, there are times when errors are made and patients do not receive the high-quality care we strive to deliver. Unfortunately, there is no "do over" of those distressing and disruptive thirty-five hours for Mr. Hanke and his wife. However, it would be shortsighted to simply lament the poor quality of care and vow to do better next time. Patient-centered health care organizations, in partnership with the affected patients and families, use incidences where errors were made (or narrowly avoided) or where patients were dissatisfied with the care provided them as a starting point to identify and rectify underlying causes of these failings. This can be accomplished by:

- Inviting patients who have experienced a medical error, near-miss, or care they considered to be of suboptimal quality to share their experiences, in person, with members of the board of directors or governing body of the organization

- Inviting these same patients/family members to sit down with the caregivers who delivered their care to share their perspective of what went wrong and how it felt for them

Of course, an organization need not wait for something to go badly to forge these partnerships with patients. Embedding ways for soliciting insights and ideas from patients and families into standard operations is a more proactive way of ensuring these important perspectives routinely inform quality improvement and strategic planning efforts. Approaches for doing so include:

- Inviting patients and family members to serve on quality and safety committees, performance improvement teams, or other standing committees—with ample support provided to them so that they can be active contributors, such as an orientation to the committee, ongoing training, assignment of a "buddy" on the committee to familiarize them to the workings and language of the group, and personal debriefs with them after their first few meetings to fill in any knowledge gaps and answer any questions

- Implementing mechanisms for patients and family members to report concerns related to care, treatment, and patient safety issues

- Establishing a patient and family advisory council that meets regularly and provides input and reactions on current practices, new initiatives, and the strategic plan/direction for the organization

- Involving patients and long-term care residents on hiring committees to understand what attributes are important from their perspective in the staff providing their care (consider, too, the message it sends to an applicant to be interviewed by a patient!)

- Conducting patient safety rounds in which staff conduct brief interviews with current patients about their perceptions of the care they are receiving and any safety concerns they may have

- Inviting patients to serve as "actors" in care delivery simulations designed to build staff competency and confidence in delivering patient-centered care

- Involving patients and family members in assessing discharge procedures to identify gaps and to develop interventions for addressing those gaps

- Engaging patient and family representatives in analyzing patient experience data and helping to develop solutions that would improve the patient experience

Getting Comfortable with Transparency

For any of these methods of engaging patients and families in improvement efforts to be constructive, they must be begun with a sincere openness to listen and learn—even when they expose things that may be unpleasant to hear. Many well-intentioned organizations invite patients to serve as patient advisers or sit on committees but then struggle with how best to engage them in a meaningful way on issues that matter to them. In fact, for many leaders, the instinct may be to sideline patient and family advisers when important issues related to quality and safety come up, dismissing them as outsiders with little understanding of how the health care system works. In fact, though, involving patients in these important dialogues and decision-making processes can reinforce human dimensions of the issues that can be easily obscured in technical and sometimes politically charged discussions. Indeed, involving patients and families who have been personally affected by a safety issue or medical error in improvement efforts can be a tremendously powerful motivator to achieve change.

Of course, the prospect of exposing an organization's flaws and system errors to patients and families can be a worrisome proposition, eliciting fears of confidentiality breaches. Having patient/family advisers sign confidentiality agreements addresses these concerns and establishes an environment of true partnership.

From Page to Practice

Review your organization's adverse event and disclosure policies and protocols, if they exist. Identify specific ways that the policies promote partnerships with patients and families, even when something unexpected occurs. Identify specific changes that could be made to further promote this spirit of partnership. For instance, are there mechanisms in place for patients to report concerns about quality and safety? Do policies address timely notification to patients (and family, as appropriate) when something unexpected occurs? Do they include guidelines for compassionate and empathetic disclosure? Do they promote involving the patient and family in understanding what occurred and determining how to prevent a recurrence? Document-specific revisions that could be incorporated into the policies to make them more patient-centered.

ENGAGING PATIENTS AND FAMILIES IN TRANSFORMING HEALTH CARE SYSTEMS

Building on the role that patients and families can play in improving quality and safety at the site level, a growing global network of patient advocates are driving improvements in health care delivery systems around the world. Initiatives such as Partnership for Patient Safety, the International Alliance of Patients' Organizations and the Health Consumer Alliance of South Australia (to name just a few) are mobilizing patients around the world to influence how care is delivered and how quality is defined on a broader scale.

A Global Network of Patient Champions: Patients for Patient Safety Programme

Bringing patients' voices to health care systems and policy, and empowering and promoting patients' engagement in patient safety initiatives worldwide has been the charge of the Patients for Patient Safety Programme (PFPS), a core pillar of the World Health Organization (WHO) Patient Safety Programme since its inception in 2004. Guided by its vision— *"Every patient receives safe health care every time and everywhere"*—the mission of the WHO Patient Safety Programme is to coordinate, facilitate, and accelerate patient safety improvements worldwide through providing global leadership; thus harnessing and facilitating the exchange of knowledge, expertise, and innovation and engaging partners and stakeholders to create sustainable changes. Aligned with this aim to engage stakeholders to create sustainable changes, PFPS is a global network of patients, health care providers, policymakers, and those affected by harm, dedicated to improving health care safety through advocacy, collaboration, and partnership.

Key to this network are "patient champions," passionate and committed individuals who share PFPS values and have completed the official PFPS capacity-building workshop, aimed at promoting dialogue between patients and policymakers and building capacity for participants to become empowered, active advocates, working in partnership with health care providers and policymakers to improve safety.

Since 2005, there have been eighteen PFPS workshops involving over six hundred participants, expanding PFPS into a global network of over 250 patient champions, thirteen collaborative organizations, and seven official in-country networks in fifty-two countries. Each individual connects to several networks at the local, national, and international levels. PFPS champions use their links to health and community stakeholders to spread the reach and impact of the program.

FIELD EXAMPLE: **CREATING CHANGE THROUGH EFFECTIVE PARTNERSHIP**

Stephanie Newell, PFPS Champion, Australia

Experiencing health care harm when her son died in the hospital was the main driver for Stephanie's work to ensure that health care practices and systems listen to, partner with, and learn from patients' experiences and take action to prevent harm to patients. Stephanie, who was present at the first Patients for Patient Safety (PFPS) workshop in London in 2005, seeks to influence change at the policy and practice levels. Having a background in the corporate sector and being cognizant to the benefits of collaboration, Stephanie works with both policymakers at the government level to develop the policy and with health care providers on the ground who implement the policy.

From organizing and facilitating the Inaugural Australian PFPS Workshop in 2009 to being a member of the Australian Commission on Safety and Quality's Expert Advisory Committee on Clinical Handover (2008–

(Continued)

2010) to presenting at Australian and international safety and quality conferences, Stephanie has facilitated regular professional education workshops for health care executives, managers, and clinicians on partnering with patients and community members for many years. Stephanie is one of the PFPS champions who have been successful in creating changes through effective partnership with health care providers and policymakers. Stephanie believes that a successful partnership must be based on a shared goal and mutual understanding. Her advice on being an effective partner is *"Inform yourself. Act professionally and demonstrate a commitment to collaboration. View yourself as a partner who brings a valuable perspective for change."*

Partnering to Improve Health Care

During the past six years, PFPS champions have made inroads in developing positive relationships with health care providers and policymakers around the world. The recent study (World Health Organization, 2010) of ninety-seven PFPS champions and its thirteen collaborating organizations indicated that positive collaboration between patients and health care providers and policymakers is key to achieving health system and policy changes. PFPS Champions represent the patient voice at policy tables, work in partnership with hospital boards, national health care quality bodies, and ministries of health to raise awareness, facilitate the implementation of WHO initiatives, and contribute to debates on policy development. Many champions influence changes through awareness-raising activities such as lecturing students, presenting at meetings and conferences, authoring publications, developing educational materials, and creating guidelines. Some focus on advocacy efforts, aimed at creating changes through policy development and implementation at institutional, national, and international levels.

MINISTRY OF HEALTH PERSPECTIVES ON ENGAGING PATIENTS

- *Kenya:* "Patient involvement is key in patient management. . . . For success we need one another. We need to gather in the country and create a forum to address patient safety issues. Through this we can put authority on its toes and get people to speak up and make us learn from mistakes."

- *Ghana:* "[PFPS] has deepened my concerns for patient safety. (Patients) provide experiential evidence that is useful for advocacy, training, and resource mobilization to advance the cause of patient safety. I have been collaborating with my fellow champions to launch the PFPS Ghana advocacy network and supporting an initiative to reduce unnecessary maternal/infant mortality."

- *Uganda:* "The workshop was a good learning exercise. I believe patients have a role to play [in] their health management, they give clear examples which can encourage involvement of other stakeholders (and) we need their cooperation. Together with my fellow PFPS Champion we have [since] been working with WHO [Uganda] to plan a conference on patient safety."

FIELD EXAMPLE: **POSITIVE COLLABORATION IN ACTION**

Nagwa Metwally, PFPS Champion, Egypt

Nagwa Metwally was one of the participants at the first Patients for Patient Safety workshop in London in 2005. As an individual with a high public

(Continued)

profile (such as being a president of the Egyptian Diplomats' Wives Association), and with connections to different groups of health care professionals, Nagwa has access to providers and policymakers at different levels.

Nagwa works at many levels and partners with many stakeholders, including patients, students, nurses, doctors, hospital management, and the Ministry of Health, in a variety of activities, ranging from lecturing and presenting to raise awareness of patient safety, to facilitating WHO initiative implementation, to raising funds for hospitals to implement the WHO Safe Surgery checklist. At the facility level, Nagwa provides feedback to hospital management regarding services, gives training on patient rights, dignity, privacy, and facilitating provider-patient relationships. She has been instrumental in the implementation of infection control measures and improved facilities in operating theatres and maternity wards at the hospital.

She is the first patient representative and the only layperson on the central hospital board that governs all hospitals and medical schools of the Ein Sham University, the second largest university of Egypt. She is also a board member of the Maternity and Gynaecology Hospital. This is also the first time that a volunteer and patient has been invited to its membership.

Nagwa's approach to advocating and promoting patient-centered care is integrity, clear communication, and teamwork: *"We must establish a clear goal,"* she says. *"Once they see that what we try to do is also in their interest, they will accept us."* On being an effective partner, she comments, *"We must be honest (to gain their trust), believe in what we say and be dedicated and serious in what we do. . . . Also we must believe in teamwork."*

In the United States, the National Strategy for Quality Improvement in Health Care is the blueprint for improving the quality of health and health care for all Americans (U.S. Department of Health and Human

Services, 2012). With a distinctly patient-centered focus, the strategy explicitly highlights the need to give individual patients and families an active role in the patient's care. This commitment to patient engagement extends beyond the point of care. It also includes partnering with patients at a national policy and reimbursement level. A nationwide initiative now links patient experiences to provider payment. Tying reimbursement directly to patients' assessments of their care experiences via Consumer Assessment of Health Care Providers and Systems (CAHPS) surveys focuses the health care system on making sure that patients and their families are true partners in preventing, diagnosing, treating, and managing illness. To ensure the National Quality Strategy meets the needs of those it is intended to benefit, a concerted effort has been made in recent years to invite patients and family members to both share their personal experiences of care and join the stakeholder groups spearheading the efforts to prioritize quality improvement efforts and identify appropriate measures of success.

Challenges

While the uptake of the patient engagement issue has increased, many challenges remain. Although many issues translate across borders and regions, different cultures and contexts mean different priorities for health care services and distinct challenges for individual patient champions (Tritter, 2009). While the approach has varied across countries, in most settings—especially low-income countries—efforts have often focused on awareness raising and establishing relationships with stakeholders. There are very few examples of successful creation, testing, and spreading of practical tools for patients to really "engage."

The level of readiness among health care providers and policymakers to embrace patient partnership also differs. Factors that motivate stakeholders to engage patients in Europe and America might differ from those in Africa or in Asia. This means that context-specific, culturally tailored approaches are necessary. Patients need to be aware, skilled, and kept abreast of current evidence and innovative advocacy efforts. Health care providers recognize the value of patients' partnership, but they need encouragement from the management and authorities to explore new and innovative approaches for services that is truly patient-centered care.

CONCLUSION: THE NEXT HORIZONS IN PATIENT ENGAGEMENT

This chapter has demonstrated the impact of patient engagement at three different levels—at the point of care, at an organizational level, and at a systems level. The next horizon in patient engagement, creating practical avenues and tools for engaging patients and their families in self-assessing, monitoring, reporting, and improving their own care, will require a multidisciplinary approach involving researchers, sociologists, civil society organizations, and engineers. This multidisciplinary, multistakeholder approach means cooperation from patient leaders, international organizations, Ministry of Health representatives, nongovernmental organizations, and civil society organizations as partners for an endeavor toward safer health care every time for every patient, everywhere.

REFERENCES

Agency for Healthcare Research and Quality. "Educating Patients Before They Leave the Hospital Reduces Readmissions, Emergency Department Visits and Saves Money." Press release, Feb. 2, 2009. Agency for Healthcare Research and Quality, Rockville, MD. www.ahrq.gov/news/press/pr2009/redpr.htm

Greene, J., and Hibbard, J. H. "Why Does Patient Activation Matter? An Examination of the Relationships Between Patient Activation and Health-Related Outcomes." *Journal of General Internal Medicine*, 2012, *27*(5), 520–526.

Institute of Medicine. *To Err Is Human: Building a Safer Health System*. Washington, DC: National Academies Press, 1999.

Longtin, Y., Sax, H., Leape, L., Sheridan, S., and others. "Patient Participation: Current Knowledge and Applicability to Patient Safety." *Mayo Proceedings*, 2010, *85*(1), 53–62.

Salzburg Global Seminar: The Greatest Untapped Resource in Healthcare? Informing and Involving Patients in Decisions About Their Medical Care, Dec. 12–17, 2010. www.Salzburgglobal.Org/Go/477

Salzburg Global Seminar: Making Health Care Better in Low and Middle Income Economies: What Are the Next Steps and How Do We Get There? Apr. 22–27, 2012. www.SalzburgGlobal.org/go/489

Tritter, J. "Revolution or Evolution: The Challenges of Conceptualizing Patient and Public Involvement in a Consumerist World." *Health Expectations*, 2009, *12*(3), 275–287.

U.S. Department of Health and Human Services. 2012 *Annual Progress Report to Congress. National Strategy for Quality Improvement in Health Care*, August 2012. Accessed Feb. 22, 2013, at www.ahrq.gov/workingforquality/nqs/ nqs2012annlrpt.pdf

World Health Organization. *Patients for Patient Safety Impact Evaluation 2010.* 2010.

11

The Role of Physicians in Patient-Centered Care

Catherine Crock, John T. Findley, Steven F. Horowitz, K. J. Lee, and Anna W. J. Omtzigt

An elderly Vietnamese woman arrived in an Emergency Department in Australia with a sudden-onset third nerve palsy. Many staff members were involved in assessing her condition. It was decided she needed an urgent brain scan. When she was told about the plan, the woman flatly refused to be taken for a scan. She repeatedly refused, said she would not have a scan, that it would only be bad and she was not going. She became quite distressed and the staff became frustrated with her. The ED director was called. She came into the room, sat down next to the patient, and took her hand. She said quietly, "Would you like me to hold your hand and walk with you to the scan?" The patient replied, "Yes, thank you" and walked to the scan room. The ED director put on a lead gown, and they held hands throughout the whole scan.

On the other side of the globe, during regular rounds on the gynecology ward, a physician met a woman who had learned the day before that she had disseminated cancer. This was the first meeting between this patient and the physician, and it was clear the news had left the patient feeling emotionally devastated. The physician asked the patient what had made her happy as a young woman and learned she had been a professional jazz singer. Within seconds she started to sing songs from her past. All the caregivers in the room fell silent, appreciating the woman's gift. She smiled and soaked up the applause. Later, the women expressed her appreciation to the physician for focusing on her talents instead of reducing her identity to that of a terminally ill patient.

—Catherine Crock, John T. Findley, Steven F. Horowitz, K. J. Lee, and Anna W. J. Omtzigt

PATIENT-CENTERED CARE: THE WORK OF THE SOUL

There are physicians who will never read this book because they feel there are more important aspects of their job that need their attention. Many may balk at the notion of reading how to be "patient-centered" when they believe they already know how to practice in this manner. After all, is there really any other way to practice medicine? In order to shift physicians' attitudes to embrace patient-centered care, perhaps we need first to understand the currently perceived role of the physician. In most countries in Western society, physicians are compensated based on volume and their success at curing illness. Thus, an environment has been created both by financial pressures and, at times, unrealistic expectations that a physician's job is to treat as many patients as possible and successfully cure them.

As a result, physicians, especially those in private practice, tend to be consumed with the nuts and bolts of delivering good patient care. For most of us, delivering good medical care has become such an all-consuming task that lengthy patient and family dialogue may be perceived as second tier in importance. With less time available to spend with a growing number of patients and a blizzard of documentation requirements, the traditional physician-patient relationship may suffer. While this result is understandable, especially as a personal survival strategy for physicians, the decrease in physician-patient face time ultimately hurts both patient and health care provider, as the healing power of positive interaction has been well documented.

Dr. David Rakel (Rakel and others, 2009, 2011) compared the recovery time and immune response of three groups of patients with upper respiratory tract infections: one group had an office visit with an empathetic physician, a second group with a decidedly unempathetic physician, and a third group with no office visit at all. Immune response was most vigorous and recovery time shortest in the group of patients who visited an empathetic physician. Of interest, recovery time was longer in the group who visited the unempathetic physician than in the group that saw no physician at all!

This research, along with the stories at the start of this chapter, illustrates that time spent being compassionate and forging human connections is time well invested—not only for the benefit of the patient and family, but also for the physicians themselves. It has been said that to serve patients rather than just "fix" them is a work of the soul, and both patient and physician are nurtured by the interaction.

As physicians with demanding and highly responsible jobs, it can be liberating to find that the more we connect on a human level with patients and families, the better the results for all concerned. The investment of time in getting to know and understand patients helps to build trust, makes patients feel more secure, and may even save time in the long run. This closer connection with patients can also contribute to our own well-being and resilience as physicians by bringing joy and fulfillment back to the workplace.

Since the early days of Planetree, a growing cadre of patient-centered physician champions has actively promoted the benefits of patient-centered care for patients, staff, and colleagues. What's more, through their daily practice, they have demonstrated what it means to be patient-centered and devised solutions for overcoming some of the most incessant barriers to practicing patient-centered care. In this chapter, five such physician champions share their insights into patient-centered care.

WHAT MATTERS MOST

From a surgical practice standpoint, the institution of universal precautions not only prevents errors and improves outcomes but also provides an opportunity to reassure patient and family. The responsible surgeon and not a surrogate should meet with the patient and family right before surgery to go over the name of the surgery and the anatomical part and precise location to be operated upon. Were these universal precautions practiced by all surgeons, many horror stories of operating on the wrong side or doing the operation on the wrong patient could be avoided. Here, best practice and patient-centered care merge to provide ideal "customer service." It is both good customer service and good quality medicine to reduce error.

Similarly, in good patient-centered care, the doctor, before prescribing any medicine, should personally double-check with the patient about any allergy to medication. It should be reiterated: doctors can be very efficient and yet render patient-centered care. While certain administrative steps can be delegated to staff or surrogates, what cannot be fully delegated is communication about the disease, the differential diagnosis, the pros and cons of alternative treatment modalities, and the risks of each therapeutic approach. These responsibilities are still the doctor's job. Helping patients grapple with life-changing illness and the search to find meaning during these critical moments remains the physician's highest calling: the physician as clinical philosopher. This is the essence of patient-centered care. It is not a new phenomenon, or a "flavor of the month" approach to care. It is simply what matters most to the patient, family, and compassionate physician.

Practicing patient-centered care is not a matter of changing the way one practices medicine, but rather changing the way one perceives and values the interactions between physician, patient, and family.

The basic tenets of patient-centered care are not rocket science from a physician's perspective. It is helpful to have educational materials in different media: print, PowerPoint, or video; but with or without them, patients appreciate doctors talking to them and annotating and drawing diagrams as needed to customize and personalize the experience. A personal follow-up phone call from the doctor is most reassuring and appreciated by patients. A powerful and transformative moment in the physician-patient relationship that exemplifies the best of patient-centered care occurs when a physician simply spends the time to listen to the patient and the patient truly feels heard.

TEN COMMANDMENTS OF PATIENT SERVICE

1. A patient is the most important person in any practice.

2. A patient is not dependent upon us . . . we are dependent on him or her.

3. A patient is not an interruption of our work . . . he or she is the purpose of it.

4. A patient does us a favor when he or she calls . . . we are not doing him or her a favor by speaking to him or her.

5. A patient is part of our business . . . not an outsider.

6. A patient is not a cold statistic . . . he or she is a flesh-and-blood human being with feelings and emotions like our own.

7. A patient is not someone to argue or match wits with.

8. A patient is one who brings us his or her needs . . . it is our job to answer those needs to the best of our ability.

9. A patient is deserving of the most courteous and attentive treatment we can give him or her.

10. Caring for patients is the reason for our jobs.

DECONSTRUCTING RESISTANCE TO PATIENT-CENTERED CARE

These commandments of patient service capture a number of universal truths about the physician-patient relationship. Certainly, this is how a doctor would want to be treated when he or she is the patient or when a loved one is unwell. Nonetheless, resistance to patient-centered care among physicians persists. This resistance can be attributed to any number of factors—misunderstanding what it means to be patient-centered or taking offense at the suggestion that one may be practicing in a way that is *not* patient-centered.

The Fear Factor

What if my patients ask for unreasonable things? What if a patient's personal beliefs and preferences are counter to evidence-based medicine? What if, by engaging with patients and family members, I am accused of having suspect professional boundaries? What if a patient reads his or her medical record and misinterprets it? What if patients and family members have more questions than I have the time to answer? What if all of this "openness" makes me more vulnerable to litigation?

These are just a few of the scenarios that may make physicians uncomfortable when they consider the effort needed to provide patient-centered care. The notion of approaching the bedside asking, "What can I do for you?" instead of, "What's wrong with you?" can feel uncomfortable—if not downright threatening—to physicians who lament the perceived loss of autonomy. In fact, though, the shift toward shared decision making does not undermine the physician's role. In a patient-centered care environment, individual needs are integrated with evidence-based information. The patient and family, along with their professional caregivers, weigh the benefits and risks of different scenarios and arrive at a collaborative approach to address individual patient preferences, needs, and values. This creates a foundation of trust and caring on which effective physician-patient relationships can flourish and where physicians can focus on *what matters most* for both parties.

The seemingly "unreasonable" patient demands or expectations dreaded by many physicians may be a result of miscommunication, inadequate or unclear information, patient and family fear, or simply a lack of personal connection or trust with the health care system. In a patient-centered approach, these difficulties become opportunities for further dialogue and education, *not* deferential acquiescence to patient or family requests.

Worth the Investment of Time

Globally, financial incentives are driving physicians to see more patients in shorter amounts of time. Yet, it is assumed that to establish rapport with patients and cultivate a collaborative approach to care takes more time (at least early on), not less. This investment of time, though, has the potential to yield higher rewards for physicians: an increase in reputation and stature, and potentially, patient volume through referrals. Paradoxically, more time spent by the physician at the front end may save time later on as patients and health care team members are better informed.

Research is limited at this time regarding how changes in patient-provider relationships *save* money. However the case for patient-centered care is clear when the conversation shifts to the costs incurred from unnecessary tests, patient and family suffering, and lost time incurred as a result of poor communication, lack of coordination of care, and lack of support for self-care (Øvretveit, 2012). Costs that could potentially be avoided when focused efforts are made to shore up patient-provider communication include avoidable readmissions, duplication in services caused by frequently changing providers, nonattendance for scheduled appointments, nonuse of dispensed medications due to patient misunderstanding, and patient safety breaches resulting from suboptimal collaboration to confirm identity, surgical site, or medication reconciliation during transitions (Øvretveit, 2012). Given these potential savings, one could reasonably argue that neither patients nor physicians can afford *not* to adopt a more patient-centered approach to care.

In the United States, the financial equation is even more clear-cut. Effective physician communication, measured by the Hospital Consumer Assessment of Healthcare Providers and System (HCAHPS) survey, will translate directly into revenue gains for hospitals.

The Need for Physician Leadership Support

Good intentions and a personal commitment to delivering patient-centered care can be stymied for even the most committed physician when faced with organizational resistance. Such institutional resistance may be fueled by the belief that patient-centered care is a "soft" endeavor that doesn't warrant the same resources and attention as, say, core measures or projects focused on safety. This line of thinking overlooks the well-documented connection between patient-centered care and overall clinical quality (Beach, Keruly, and Moore, 2006; DiMatteo, 1994; DiMatteo, Sherbourne and others, 1993; Fremont and others, 2001; Greenfield and others, 1988; Kim, Kaplowitz, and Johnston, 2004; Little and others, 2001; Meterko and others, 2010; Stewart and others, 2000). Physicians who become outspoken patient-centered care champions for their organizations are the standard-bearers for a course of action that will influence quality, operations, service, and financial performance. Most important, when a group of physician champions joins forces to advance the cause of patient-centered care, they become change agents and may provide the impetus for significant cultural transformation throughout the organization.

The most effective physician leaders are able to help employees build a collective picture of how care can be delivered. They appeal to the creativity of all professionals and are respected catalysts for transformation when passionately embracing principles of patient-centered care. They encourage other professional caregivers to find ways to fulfill the needs of their patients and to work in harmony with their colleagues. Physician leaders participating on patient-centered care committees and task forces ensure the physician's unique perspective remains part of the dialogue and planning while reinforcing patient-centered care as an organizational aim that touches all stakeholders.

Patient-centered physician leaders embody the principles of compassionate patient care and have a unique platform, often providing the sole voice of the patient and family during leadership meetings. An underpinning of any patient-centered culture is that all staff members are caregivers who have the ability to influence the patient experience, directly or indirectly. Physician leaders who forge connections with colleagues from many different disciplines and departments demonstrate, through their actions, that patient-centered care is a great equalizer. Successful implementation of patient-centered care requires that caregivers from all departments and disciplines collaborate for the sake of the patient. Organizations need physicians to identify and help break down the walls of entrenched organizational silos and take risks in seeking out and understanding different perspectives. Accordingly, patient-centered physician champions must go out of their way not only to be approachable, but to proactively approach other health care workers for the common good.

TACKLING THE CHALLENGE OF THE DISRESPECTFUL PHYSICIAN

Although in theory physicians are unified by their desire to take care of the ill in a compassionate manner, the stressors inherent in the daily practice of medicine may, at times, pit well-intentioned goals against the fragility of interpersonal interactions. The same desire that fuels passion to care for others can spill over into inappropriate aggression toward others if egos are allowed to get in the way. There is a fine line between an appropriately matched passion for what one does and inappropriate and abusive behavior toward other health care workers. Acting in service to others is driven by one's passion to care for the sick. Acting out toward others is driven by stress, frustration, fatigue, and poor coping mechanisms and communication skills. Older physicians may cling to a more paternalistic system that has been replaced by a team approach and dialogue.

Historically, our culture has been overly tolerant of the occasional outburst toward a staff member or patient by a tired or frustrated physician, as if it is simply one of the costs of practicing medicine. In essence, we have grown accustomed to a culture that favors physician privilege and autonomy. In the past there may have been different rules of behavior and more tolerance for physicians with large practices or hard-to-replace skills. Although this may have been acceptable at one time, it has been demonstrated that the rapport established between the physician and other staff members, good or bad, has far-reaching implications for the patient being cared for (Leape and others, 2012). Recent data suggests that disrespectful behavior toward staff or peers has an impact on the recipient's ability to think clearly in the clinical setting, ultimately inhibiting his or her ability to make sound clinical judgments at the point of care. Additional data suggests that physicians who are allowed to act in this way tend to demonstrate an underlying resistance to collaboration with others and to following procedures known to improve patient safety (Weng, 2008).

Although it has traditionally been more "acceptable" for physicians to demonstrate disrespectful behavior than other health care workers, one could make a compelling argument that if physicians, as a group, truly intend to demonstrate concern for the patient, they must cooperate and become role models for creating a culture that extols the virtue of temperance and dialogue to resolve disagreements.

In the ideal setting, conflict would be approached as an opportunity to reach out to a peer that may be struggling or is simply unaware of the impact that his or her disrespectful behavior has on the patient experience. In reality, the typical response has been to simply ignore these outbursts in order to avoid exacerbating the situation. More and more health care organizations are drawing a line in the sand with a "zero tolerance" policy for the disruptive physician. In many cases, a disruptive physician's actions may originate from a perception that he or she is the only person who really cares enough about the patient to aggressively prevent harm. Coming from this egocentric mind-set, anything done to protect the patient seems justified, even if it involves abusive behavior or bullying. This type of behavior may lead to a reluctance on the part of a colleague or team member to voice a potentially important opinion, an effect well described as a cause of airline pilot error and physician error.

Choosing to ignore disrespectful behavior simply sends the message that this type of behavior is acceptable within the organization. It is the collective responsibility of the organizational leaders, peer leadership, and front-line staff to cultivate a culture that demonstrates understanding, elevates awareness, and establishes the expectation of mutual respect regardless of circumstance.

According to Dr. Leape of the Harvard School of Public Health, in order to eliminate disrespectful behavior a cultural transformation must occur that establishes a supportive and nurturing environment with high levels of mutual interpersonal trust, interpersonal responsibility, person centeredness, supportiveness for coworkers, civility, friendliness, and creativity (Leape, 2012).

It is assumed that to be a physician is to be a leader. In truth, this is a skill that is not explicitly taught during physicians' many years of training, but becomes implicit as physicians mature in their practice. In the past, we physicians led by default, our words often going unchallenged, at times to the detriment of the patient. In the current era the team approach has taken over, and the physician may or may not retain this traditional role as leader. The hallmark of a physician leader is to demonstrate equanimity at all times, maintaining a calm composure and evenness of temper in stressful situations. True leaders may or may not be born with the power to inspire, but the "magic" of leadership occurs in partnership with colleagues. It is a by-product of a group process in which an individual's sense of shared social identity enables him or her to exert influence over others. In order to elevate a disrespectful peer to a higher standard of care and gain the interpersonal skills needed for leadership, health care institutions must artfully integrate counseling, training, personal history, hopes, and values into a code of ethics that inspires physicians to represent and achieve these goals and thus to lead.

From Page to Practice

It is likely that from time to time, most of us have manifested elements of disrespectful behavior that have interfered with our ability to be physician leaders. Are you a disrespectful physician? Ask yourself these questions:

- Do you seek to control those around you and particularly those junior to you in order to further your position?
- Do you refuse to listen to the views and opinions of those you consider to be beneath you in the system?
- Do you treat your colleagues with respect at all times?
- Do you undermine colleagues who present views that are different from your own?
- Do you try to use the force of your will to get your own way?
- Do you teach by humiliation or ridicule?
- Do you include people beneath you in decision making?
- Do you readily accept feedback on how your behavior is perceived?
- Do you misuse your power to further your own ambition?
- Do you withhold information from other staff or patients/family as a way of maintaining power and control?

THE PHYSICIAN PERSPECTIVE ON . . .

Planetree promotes a number of patient-centric practices designed to address the full range of patient and family needs and preferences. These hallmark practices have arisen out of patient and family focus group feedback regarding what matters most to them. When it comes to what matters most, surveys commonly show different priorities between physician and patient/family perspectives. In this section, we address some common physician concerns about specific patient-centered practices.

Complementary and Alternative Medicine (CAM)

Many physicians are closed off to the concept of complementary or alternative approaches to care and may not even accept peer-reviewed, evidence-based approaches in this area. In one memorable staff meeting at which the hospital presented its plan to create an evidence-based center for integrative medicine, a well-respected senior physician addressed his fellow physicians by saying: "Are we going to allow voodoo medicine into this hospital?" Nonetheless, health care consumers' interest in pursuing a variety of unconventional treatment modalities is well described. Professional caregivers who do not work in partnership with patients to understand the full scope of treatment modalities already being utilized get an incomplete picture of the patients' health status and may put the patients at risk by not understanding the potential risks of prescribing allopathic pharmaceuticals together with unknown supplements.

The Planetree model promotes patient choice and access to a variety of treatment modalities, including those characterized as complementary or alternative, such as massage therapy, Reiki, acupuncture, healing touch, and naturopathy when there are no medical contraindications to their use. However, the Planetree approach is not prescriptive about specifically *what* modalities to offer. If the goal is to be responsive to the needs, interests, and preferences of health care consumers, then a first step is to explore with patients what modalities they are currently using or are interested in learning more about. Physicians must be engaged in this effort and learn what patients are doing and taking on their own.

Physicians must develop opinions based upon available evidence about the risks and benefits of nonallopathic approaches. Early adopters or champions of complementary therapies can be enlisted to impart their experience and knowledge, and to solicit feedback from patients on the effects they experienced to share with colleagues. For instance, in the years following the introduction of the integrative medical center cited previously, the integrative physicians diffused anxiety about "voodoo medicine" by sending comprehensive consultation reports back to the primary care doctors explaining potentially dangerous interactions between common supplements and prescribed medications such as fish oil, St. John's wort, and warfarin. Also, prescribing low-risk diet and lifestyle options for patients with chronic inflammation-based conditions along with cited references for the referring physician may add to the knowledge within the medical community.

In the spirit of providing access to information so that health care consumers can make informed choices about their care, individual providers and organizations are encouraged to make information about CAM modalities available, as well as to establish a referral base for those modalities known to be of interest to their patients.

Although we believe we are fulfilling our obligation of "first do no harm" to the best of our abilities, if we are not fully conversant with the CAM evidence-based literature, we may be missing the opportunity to prescribe relatively inexpensive, low-risk remedies for a variety of chronic diseases.

A prime example of this is the under utilization of post–myocardial infarction cardiac rehabilitation. Hammill, Curtis, Schulman, and Whellan (2010) have demonstrated a dose-response relationship between the number of cardiac rehabilitation visits and four-year survival, with a remarkable 47 percent reduction in death rate for patients completing all thirty-six sessions versus those attending only once. Of the more than eighteen thousand patients surveyed, fewer than one in five patients ever went to cardiac rehabilitation, and of these only 18 percent completed all thirty-six sessions. This information suggests that were more physicians familiar with positive outcome of cardiac rehabilitation data and strongly recommended it to their patients, improved outcomes might be expected.

Open Disclosure

Open, bidirectional communication is at the heart of patient-centered care. This emphasis on transparency and openness does not lessen when something unexpected or problematic occurs; in fact, it becomes all the more important. Many health care organizations have centralized the way they handle complaints in the interest of expediting resolution. With a focus on partnership and relationship building in a patient-centered environment of care, it is advisable that complaints be handled by the health care team itself, with support as necessary from complaint officers. This ensures that the professionals involved understand firsthand from the patient or family member(s) their perspectives on what happened and that they are informed about the impact of the (mis)communication. When addressed early on in a forthcoming, transparent manner by those directly involved, effective two-way communication can be restored. What's more, because complications of treatment are inevitable and large litigation payments can erode already thin hospital margins, the fact that a patient or family who has experienced open and honest communication following an adverse event is less likely to lodge a formal complaint or lawsuit represents both a solid ethical and financial strategy.

WHY OPEN DISCLOSURE MAKES A DIFFERENCE

Following the death of their father who passed away in the hospital, a family had questions and concerns about the care he received. He had been found next to his bed, and his family wanted to know the details of what happened in the last hours of their father's life. Their complaint was forwarded to an official central committee responsible for handling complaints. The patient's medical records were reviewed and the information passed on to the family members in a series of three formal meetings. Unfortunately, these measures fell short of answering their questions. For more than six months, the family grieved.

Eventually the director of the medical board became aware of the situation, met with the family, and devised a plan to get the answers the family sought. A meeting was arranged with the family members and the nurses who were working on the floor the night their father died. The health care professionals shared with the family members how their father spent his last hours. They told them the medical details and, more meaningful to the family, they shared how he felt, what he ate, and how he was prepared for the night. The family members were impressed by the caring attitudes of the nurses. In a single meeting, their need for detailed information about their father's last hours was fulfilled in a way that the three prior meetings had failed to do. At the completion of their discussion with the nurses, the family withdrew their formal complaint.

Shared Medical Record

Creating partnerships and opening up dialogue between patients and physicians requires a breaking down of the barriers between the highly educated health care professionals providing treatment and the very vulnerable human beings who entrust these professionals with their care. Facilitating patients' access to the medical record is a key strategy for breaking down those barriers. Doing so not only stimulates discussion about treatment, health goals, and lifestyle changes, but also reassures patients that nothing is being kept from them—that they are, in every respect, integral members of their care teams. Sharing the record is an opportunity for teaching, answering questions, and true and open dialogue that is likely to lower patient and family "serum paranoia levels." Realizing these aims requires the involvement of health care professionals to help patients understand their record. It is useful for a health care worker to be available to clarify medical phrases that may be misinterpreted, such as "end-stage renal disease." For more on the Shared Medical Record, see Chapter Five.

IF YOU'RE NOT PART OF THE SOLUTION, YOU'RE PART OF THE PROBLEM

The concept of "if you're not part of the solution then you're part of the problem," a common slogan in the 1960s, pertains here. Even small changes may go a long way toward improving the situation. During a Planetree visit to a Veteran's Administration hospital, physicians were asked to identify a single facet of their practice they could change that would enhance the experience of their patients. One physician responded by saying that he regularly attends clinic at the hospital, but on Thursdays he has to leave in time to make a regularly scheduled 5 p.m. appointment. The result of this was that the last two patients of the day commonly did not get his full attention. The physician's commitment to change was simply to move his regularly scheduled appointment from 5 p.m. to 6 p.m. so that the last two patients of the day got the time and thoughtfulness they deserved. When each physician examines his or her own practice and chooses to make even a simple change in favor of the patient, the cumulative effect of hundreds of such changes can shift the culture of an entire organization. The impact of an entire medical staff making many small adjustments can produce a cultural sea change throughout a hospital that enhances both the physicians' and patients' experience and can even have a ripple effect on the entire community.

From Page to Practice

Ask yourself the same questions: "What single facet of my practice could I change to that would enhance the experience of my patients? What would it take for me to make this change?"

CONCLUSION: PERSONAL COMMITMENTS PHYSICIANS CAN MAKE TO BE MORE PATIENT-CENTERED

- Endeavor to make health care interactions humane and healing experiences for patients, families, and other staff.

- Endeavor to build and sustain trusting, loving, supportive relationships at work.

- Connect person to person, with integrity, toward everyone you work with to get the best out of each interaction. Model this behavior to other staff.

- Endeavor to inspire others by demonstrating the value you place on compassion, good communication, commitment, collaboration, and creativity on a daily basis.

- Endeavor to behave in a noncompetitive, nurturing, and generous way.

- A nonjudgmental attitude is vital.

- A can-do attitude makes a difference and is infectious. Encourage staff you work with to continually think of ways to improve the experience of patients, families, and other staff.

- If there are administrative barriers or rules, question whether they are there to benefit the organization rather than the patients and families. Help staff think creatively about other ways to solve the problem.

- If we can't say yes to a reasonable patient request, question whether it is a system or administrative barrier that could be relaxed or changed to allow the request to be fulfilled.

- Encourage your patients and families to give feedback. Ensure that it is acted upon.

- Mentor junior doctors and other staff and give them latitude to use their ideas and creativity.

- Ask your colleagues: What would be one thing in your daily work that you would like to change to improve the patient experience?

- Network with like-minded physicians. Form a group that meets regularly to discuss patient- and family-centered care and support each other.

- Explain to patients and families that they are part of the team, helping to improve care for their loved ones, and make that care safer. Let them know that their expertise will be listened to and valued.

By investing the effort to restore the time-honored and sacred physician-patient relationship as best as possible in today's tumultuous medical world, we will not only relieve suffering and enhance healing for our patients, but also for ourselves.

REFERENCES

Beach, M. C., Keruly, J., and Moore, R. D. "Is the Quality of the Patient-Provider Relationship Associated with Better Adherence and Health Outcomes for Patients with HIV?" *Journal of General Internal Medicine*, 2006, *21*(6), 661–665.

Dimatteo, M. R. "Enhancing Patient Adherence to Medical Recommendations." *JAMA*, 1994, *271*(1), 79–83.

Dimatteo, M. R., Sherbourne, C. D., Hays, R. D., Ordway, L., and others. "Physicians' Characteristics Influence Patients' Adherence to Medical Treatment: Results from the Medical Outcomes Study." *Health Psychology*, 1993, *12*(2), 93–102.

Fremont, A. M., Cleary, P. D., Hargraves, J. L., Rowe, R. M., and others. "Patient-Centered Processes of Care and Long-Term Outcomes of Acute Myocardial Infarction." *Journal of General Internal Medicine*, 2001, *16*(12), 800–808.

Greenfield, S., Kaplan, H. S., Ware, J. E. Jr., Yano, E. M., and others. "Patients' Participation in Medical Care: Effects on Blood Sugar Control and Quality of Life in Diabetes." *Journal of General Internal Medicine*, 1988, *3*(5), 448–457.

Hammill, B. G., Curtis, L. H., Schulman, K. A., and Whellan, D. J. "Relationship Between Cardiac Rehabilitation and Long-Term Risks of Death and Myocardial Infarction Among Elderly Medicare Beneficiaries." *Circulation*, 2010, *121*(1), 63–70.

Kim, S. S., Kaplowitz, S., and Johnston, M. V. "The Effects of Physician Empathy on Patient Satisfaction and Compliance." *Evaluation and the Health Professions*, 2004, *27*(3), 237–251.

Leape, L. L., Shore, M. F., Dienstag, J. L., Mayer, R. J., and others. "Perspective: A Culture of Respect, Part 1 and Part 2: The Nature and Causes of Disrespectful Behavior by Physicians." *Academic Medicine*, 2012, *87*(7), 845–858.

Little, P., Everitt, H., Williamson, I., Warner, G., and others. "Observational Study of Effect of Patient Centredness and Positive Approach on Outcomes of General Practice Consultations." *BMJ*, 2001, *323*(7318), 908–11.

Meterko, M., Wright, S., Lin, H., Lowy, E., and others. "Mortality Among Patients with Acute Myocardial Infarction: The Influences of Patient-Centered Care and Evidence-Based Medicine." *Health Services Research,* 2010, *45*(5), 1188–1204.

Øvretveit, J. *Do Changes to Patient-Provider Relationships Improve Quality and Save Money? Vol. 1: Summary of a Review of the Evidence.* London: Health Foundation, 2012. www.Health.Org.Uk

Rakel, D., Barrett, B., Zhang, Z., Hoeft, T., and others. "Perception of Empathy in the Therapeutic Encounter: Effects on the Common Cold." *Patient Education and Counseling,* 2011, *85*(3), 390–397.

Rakel, D. P., Hoeft, T. J., Barrett, B. P., Chewning, B. A., and others. "Practitioner Empathy and the Duration of the Common Cold." *Family Medicine,* 2009, *41*(7), 494–501.

Stewart, M., Brown, J. B., Donner, A., Mcwhinney, I. R., and others. "The Impact of Patient-Centered Care on Outcomes." *Journal of Family Practice,* 2000, *49*(9), 796–804.

Weng, H. C. "Does the Physician's Emotional Intelligence Matter? Impacts of the Physician's Emotional Intelligence on the Trust, Patient-Physician Relationship, and Satisfaction." *Health Care Management Review,* 2008, *33*(4), 280–288.

12

Creating a Patient-Centered Continuum of Care

Michelle Bowman, Sylvie Doiron, Deborah Felsenthal, Joep P. Koch, Marci Nielsen, and Heidi Ruis

Just two and a half weeks after being discharged from the hospital to a nursing home, my father, who has congestive heart failure, had to be go back to the hospital. Just eighteen days earlier, he had left the hospital with a packet of instructions of warning signs to look out for, information on medications, and instructions for taking care of himself. My mother died six years ago, and I'm his only daughter. I live three hours away and was unable to be there when he left the hospital. I called him shortly after he arrived at the nursing home and asked him about what the doctors and nurses had to say about his heart and what lifestyle changes he would need to make, like diet and exercise. He did his best to reassure me that he would be okay, but I could tell he was having a hard time remembering everything the doctors and nurses had told him. He recalled the nurse at the hospital telling him that he would need to check his daily weight so that he would be alert to any weight gain. He was even given a log for tracking his weight. By the time he got settled in at the nursing home, it seemed he had completely forgotten about the weight log. I think he expected

that the aides caring for him were keeping an eye on his weight. After all, they were weighing him frequently—a few times a week at least. The dietician at the hospital gave him a stern talking-to about eating only low-salt foods, and even provided him with some recipes for healthy meals she guaranteed wouldn't taste "healthy." At the nursing home, I know he did his best to follow the dietician's guidelines, but he told me that sometimes it wasn't clear to him on the menu in the dining room which foods he could and couldn't have. Before leaving the hospital, he was also instructed to see his primary care physician for a follow-up appointment. My father and I had both been assured that the nursing home had a physician who was available to provide care for all of its residents. He made an appointment with that physician, but unfortunately was readmitted to the hospital for congestive heart failure the day before he was to meet with the doctor.
—Sonya

Implied within the term itself, *patient-centered care* is care organized around the experiences and needs of the patient. These experiences and needs are not isolated to one moment in time, nor to a specific provider or care setting—not even to a single disease or diagnosis. Given this, it is shortsighted to reduce the "patient experience" to just the most recent hospitalization, diagnostic test, or home care visit. To deliver comprehensive patient-centered care, the health care experience—and the person at the center of it—must be considered in their totality, with an appreciation and understanding of the complexity and multidimensionality of *that particular* patient's experience.

Nonetheless, in many health care delivery systems, fragmentation continues to be the norm, more so than integration and coordination. According to the Institute of Medicine, lack of care coordination can be unsafe, and even fatal, when abnormal test results are not communicated correctly, prescriptions from multiple doctors conflict with each other, or primary care physicians do not receive hospital discharge plans for their patients (Meyers and others, 2010). Moreover, lack of coordination adds to the cost of care due to duplicated services, preventable hospital readmissions, and overuse of more intensive procedures. Certainly, it is not unreasonable to suggest that Sonya's father's story would have unfolded differently were effective care coordination measures in place.

From Page to Practice

As a team, review the case of a patient or resident who was readmitted to the hospital. Debrief what could have worked better and where the breakdowns in communication occurred. What could be done differently in the future?

True patient-centered care transcends the silos that frustrate providers and patients alike and undermine the delivery of optimal care. Taking cues from the patient experience, a patient-centered continuum of care extends beyond a single setting or discrete episode of care. It emphasizes coordination, continuity, collaboration, and communication. It promotes a team approach to the management of chronic conditions. Its responsibility goes beyond caring for the ill and infirm to managing the health and wellness of the population.

For many communities and health care delivery systems, this vision of a patient-centered continuum of care is one to aspire to. And indeed, there have never been greater incentives to convert the aspiration into reality. Global trends in health care reform focus on curbing costs and enhancing quality. Comprehensive reform will not be achieved if these aims are approached disjointedly by individual institutions. What it will take is a collective and cooperative effort across the care continuum to facilitate more seamless transitions, maximize efficiencies across settings and providers, and activate patients to become more effective managers of their own health and wellness goals.

Indeed, some of the health care systems that have reputations as the best in the world are grounded in a "cradle to grave" approach to care in which care coordination and population health management are fundamental drivers of quality. As a global community of health care leaders invested in reorienting provider- and setting-centered care to a more patient-centered approach, we can learn from these systems that serve as examples of how to create a patient-centered continuum.

LESSONS FROM THE FIELD: THE NETHERLANDS

The Dutch health care system is organized around "care lines." The first care line, encompassing family doctors (GPs), preventive health care, home health care, and visiting nurses, is the "gatekeeper" of the second care line, which includes all forms of hospitals (acute care, psychiatric, and rehabilitation), nursing homes, hospice care, and residential care.

Although there is considerable cooperation within this system, transitioning between care lines and payers can nonetheless present challenges. To address these, in 1995, the team at Rivas Zorggroep, a large, integrated health care system based out of Gorinchem, endeavored to redesign its vast system in such a way that patients could easily transition across care lines. At the time, patients often experienced delays for needed care due to waiting lists. Hospitals (triggered by the insurance companies) were pushing to get patients out of their expensive beds. Capacity issues resulted in individuals with dementia remaining at home as they waited to move into a residential care center where they would get the more intensive care they needed. In other cases, the discharge of a rehabilitation patient eager to go home may be delayed due to a shortage in home health care staff.

Guided by the goals to simplify these transitions, improve quality and access to care, and enhance patient satisfaction, the system implemented a series of changes which have resulted in better care for patients, fewer hospitalizations and nursing home admissions, and subsequently reduced costs. The steps taken to achieve these outcomes include:

- *Adoption of a team approach.* As the Rivas team embarked on this journey to create a patient-centered continuum, staff from all types of care were placed in groups. The main goal was for the staff to get to know each other, to examine the factors at the root of the system's malfunctions, and to analyze the problem of patients not getting the care they needed while having to wait.

- *Creation of a centralized patient transfer unit (PlanService).* Equipped with up-to-date information on the capacity of every site within the system (versus capacity being managed at the local level), this unit is able to manage a patient's care and movement across care lines through a variety of consecutive services, from discharge from the hospital, admission to a nursing home, and then a return home with home care services.

- *Coordination of transitions.* Staff across the system familiarized themselves with each other's processes and challenges, specifically around discharges and transitions. Today, there are shared pathways that contain the best practices for various types of patient care across settings. Hospitals, nursing homes, rehabilitation, and home health care share a responsibility to create a continuum of care for the patient. For instance, patients who have undergone total hip replacements are supplied with information and training in advance of hospitalization about what they may expect in the various stages of their treatment. In the rehabilitation unit of the nursing home, family members are trained to support the patient at home so they know what they can do and how they can help. Therapists analyze the patient's home situation and suggest adjustments for comfort and safety. They will make sure the patient's home is ready for his or her arrival.

- *Enhancement of care coordination with home health care workers in the community.* The role of Rivas home health care workers is to arrange care for patients at their homes and to communicate with the patient's GP. When specialized care is needed, the home health care worker calls in a specialized professional (nurse, therapist, and sometimes even a doctor) from the Rivas Network. When a patient is discharged from the hospital to their home, the specialized nurse from the ward gets in contact with a home health care nurse from the patient's region. Together they arrange the best follow-up procedures for the patient and communicate with the community's GP group. The Rivas home health care professional also cooperates with other organizations within the community, like churches, volunteers, housing organizations, police, and so on, in order to get all factors that are needed for the best care in one line of cooperation for the benefit of the patient. Rivas has also a special program for frail elderly patients to keep them stable and safely and comfortably living at home for as long as possible. In some cases, help is provided up to six different times a day.

- *Introduction of a new patient information system.* The electronic patient dossier (EPD) enhances coordination and communication among multiple caregivers within the system treating the same patient. Rivas approaches this in such a way that the ownership of information is entirely in the hands of the patient. This forces the professionals to communicate with the patient in such a way that information is meaningful and comprehensible.

LESSONS FROM THE FIELD: QUEBEC

Financed through fifty years of taxpayer contributions, the public health and social services system in Quebec is responsible for providing accessible, continuous, and quality services. The organization of services in Quebec is performed on a local, regional, and provincial basis in a hierarchical model of care that encourages collaborative work and enhanced sharing of responsibilities. Key components of the strategy to achieve this coordinated approach include:

- *Centralized health and social services centers* (CSSS) that are responsible for the coordination of all public and private services in their communities, from preventive measures to alternatives when care can no longer reestablish a person's full autonomy.

- *Patient navigators* or case managers who act as guides into the network for patients, families, and loved ones.

- *Consortium or network of services* for different kind of conditions.

- The development of *individualized intervention or service plans* that define with each individual patient their objectives, procedures and those responsible for them, expected results, and when the plan will be reevaluated. The plan constitutes an efficient method of ensuring continuity of services and avoiding duplication. Part of the role of the patient navigator is to ensure that the plan is discussed with all those concerned and that it will be followed and adapted according to changes in the person's condition.

- *Clinical-administrative information technology systems that facilitate the transfer of information* relevant to each person's situation and a history of care and services. These systems enable a truly integrated network of care and services for people experiencing a loss of autonomy due to aging. Similar systems have been implemented or are being developed for those with complex or chronic conditions. An electronic health care file system on a grand scale will allow all citizens to access essential information about their particular health care program on the same platform as doctors and other stakeholders through secure Internet connections accessible throughout Quebec. This project is currently being tested in four regions of the province.

Through laws and regulations, existing structures, and approaches and measures guiding care and clinical tools required by service providers, Quebec is a testament to the priority accorded to continuity of care and services provided in a participatory manner that empowers patients and their loved ones. Continuity of care and services is important to ensure health care network efficiency, but above all to provide a secure and pleasant experience for people.

STRATEGIES FOR IMPROVING CONTINUITY

Despite these success stories, a study of the experiences of chronically and seriously ill patients in eleven countries concluded that gaps in care coordination and transitions between hospitals and other community-based settings, communication lapses between specialists and primary care physicians, and delays in receiving test results were evident in every country surveyed (Schoen and others, 2011). More than half of Germans (56 percent) and French (53 percent) patients and more than two in five Norwegian (43 percent) and U.S. (42 percent) patients reported gaps in care coordination, including duplicate tests being ordered, medical records or test results not being available during a medical appointment, or providers not sharing important information with each other. In contrast, only 20 percent of U.K. patients and 23 percent of Swiss patients reported such gaps in care (Schoen and others, 2011).

Narrowing the Gaps

By their very nature, transitions involve multiple entities, which means that any effective solutions for coordination must reach beyond any one site or setting. For this reason, many approaches focus on equipping the patient—as the most obvious source of continuity across care settings—with tools to manage and coordinate their own care. Examples include:

- *Medication lists* which serve as a personal record of current medications a patient is taking

- *Personal health records*, or a centralized location where patients compile and track information about their health and health care needs

- *Coaching* for patients and their informal caregivers to enable them to effectively manage their care

- *Printed discharge instructions* provided on transition to another care setting and written in a language the patient will understand

- *Follow-up calls* after transition to the next setting of care to reinforce important next steps (such as making follow-up appointments) and reassess comprehension of discharge instructions

FIELD EXAMPLE: **SUPPORTING COMMUNITY-BASED, PATIENT-CENTERED TRANSITIONS OF CARE**

Longmont United Hospital, Longmont, Colorado, USA

At Longmont United Hospital (LUH), a not-for-profit community-based 201-bed hospital in Colorado, a multifaceted Transitions of Care program has been introduced with the goal of minimizing the economic impact of readmissions on the health system, and reducing the physical and psychological impact of readmissions on patients' well-being. Key strategies in LUH's Transitions of Care Model include:

- Registered nurse champions, role modeling, and teaching transitions of care strategies on a daily basis
- Utilization of evidence-based tools to assess patient activation and readiness for change
- Development of a Transition of Care Plan which emphasizes patient-identified health care goals and needs
- Weekly multidisciplinary team meetings to break down silos
- Innovative therapeutic interventions, including integrative/whole person care
- Increased utilization of technology, including iPads, with online surveys to increase patient engagement and confidence in interacting with their physicians and other health care providers

FROM THE INPATIENT SETTING TO THE COMMUNITY SETTING

Acknowledging that an acute care hospitalization is a challenging time in a patient's experience to teach and change health behaviors, Longmont United Hospital has made a focused effort to expand upon its Transitions of Care program by developing additional interventions for the community setting. At the heart of the Transitions of Care program is a team of community volunteers known as Care Partners. A Care Partner is a volunteer

(Continued)

recruited, trained, and matched to work in a peer support relational manner with patients who have experienced frequent hospital admissions. By complementing other aspects of the Transitions of Care program with support from Care Partners, LUH has been able to provide a more personalized and patient-centered approach to working with patients readmitted to the hospital.

The hospital has also turned its attention to engaging and evaluating community members to determine their needs and goals *before* they are ever hospitalized. Through LUH's outpatient senior wellness program, a Patient Activation Measure tool is administered, providing the opportunity to engage community members in a discussion of their health and wellness needs outside of a hospitalization episode. Wellness clinics and wellness RN coaches are available to support community members in maintaining their health. Classes promote behavior change in a setting that is peer-based, wellness-focused, and confidence-building. The classes are shifting away from a lecture style of teaching into a more interactive and engaged model. Additional components of LUH's community-based and patient-centered Transitions of Care model are:

- Interactive inpatient group classes on diabetes management and congestive heart failure (bringing three or more patients together is more cost-effective and increases participation and patient activation than previous one-on-one teaching methods)

- Presurgical orthopedic group teaching classes to promote knowledge about postsurgical healing, while also providing peer support and camaraderie

- A weekly meditation class for inpatients, community members, and hospital staff

- Monthly "Get to Know Us/You" community health orientation class to meet new community members and introduce them to wellness programs

- Monthly community-based Advanced Directives planning in group setting (for example, one married senior couple who'd known each other since age twelve applied a technique to encourage "the conversation" and said they discovered things they'd never discussed before)

- Programs to encourage self-care, such as "Medications and You: Who's in Charge?"

- Collaborating with other community groups/organizations—for example, Farmers' Market, LiveWell Longmont—to make connections, share the stories, avoid duplication of effort

- Presentations to community service groups to increase awareness of health care issues

Patient-Centered Primary Care

As this field example illustrates, community collaboration and strategic partnerships are essential for tackling the challenge of creating a patient-centered continuum of care. These partnerships must extend to primary care providers. Improved care coordination is emerging as an essential role of the primary care provider, especially for those patients with multiple ongoing health care needs that cannot be met by a single clinician or organization (Harman and others, 2010).

The Patient-Centered Medical Home as the Hub of Care Coordination

The patient-centered medical home (PCMH) is steadily gaining traction as an effective and efficient primary care–based health system that produces better patient health outcomes at lower costs than traditional care. The PCMH emphasizes providing primary care through partnership with patients that is comprehensive, coordinated, and accessible. Through a PCMH, patients receive improved preventive care and chronic condition management that results in improved patient outcomes and a reduction of redundant or unnecessary and expensive visits, tests, and procedures.

The PCMH accomplishes this goal in large part due to its commitment to and emphasis on patient-centered care coordination. The PCMH coordinates and tracks all aspects of a patient's health care both within its own walls and through the medical neighborhood, serving as a true "home base" for its patients. Proper patient-centered care coordination ensures both that the medical home is at the center of the medical neighborhood, and that the patient is at the center of her medical home. It addresses the patient as a whole, not as one sick part; it takes into consideration her medical, social, developmental, behavioral, educational, and financial background in order to optimize health and wellness outcomes.

Begins with the Patient, a Care Plan, and the Care Team Creating a patient-centered continuum of care requires a team that is committed to addressing the needs of the patient and their families. In the initial stages of transitioning to improved care coordination, having *set, agreed-on health goals developed by the patient and her primary care clinician* provides a useful reference point for the care team. Oriented toward the patient's preferences, this care plan provides the care team with a "map" that allows for standardization of protocols, medication management, and can assist in streamlining communications across the medical neighborhood, including medical specialists, psychologists, and physical therapists. At each visit, during a previsit interview with a nurse or medical assistant, the patient should be asked about any possible updates since her last visit, such as specialist visits or medication changes.

Patient feedback is vital at this early stage as well. Patients should work with the care team to establish a method of communication that works well for them, and establish when and how they should be contacted, and how they should contact the PCMH with questions or concerns, taking into account any cultural, language, developmental, or other barriers that may prevent proper communication with the care team. Patients can benefit from having access to an *online patient portal,* allowing for simple requests, such as appointment or refill requests, to be fulfilled automatically, while also having a way to access their personal health records and contact their providers. For patients uncomfortable or unable to use an online portal, other methods of communication, such as having *24/7 access to telephonic services,* should be available.

Using Electronic Health Records Another critical means of ensuring care coordination within the PCMH and across the medical neighborhood is through the use of electronic health records (EHR). Electronic health records store and transmit health information among various types of health care providers and are increasingly important in maintaining continuity of care as they allow for structured organization and evaluation of patient data and easy transfer of patient records. As EHR systems become operational, with the ability to exchange demographic and clinical information across health systems, their use will empower the care team to use data to measure and track performance of health care quality and population health outcomes.

FIELD EXAMPLE: **PROVENHEALTH NAVIGATOR**

ProvenHealth Navigator, the PCMH of Pennsylvania-based Geisinger Health System, tracks metrics on real-time data gathered from its EHR system in order to determine and evaluate quality outcomes in fields such as patient and physician satisfaction and chronic disease care. The results are significant: for its commercially insured ProvenHealth Navigator patients, Geisinger found a 37.9 percent reduction in hospital admissions since joining the PCMH, and a 28 percent reduction for its Medicare patients (Steele and others, 2010).

Care Coordination Concepts Care coordination in the PCMH requires not only coordination with itself and outside practitioners, but also coordinating care within its own walls. At the start of each workday, many PCMHs rely on a *daily huddle,* in which all members of the care team gather to review the schedule, and discuss issues with patients and how to resolve problems. The schedule they work with must contain *open slots for patients who need same-day appointments,* so that nobody will need to be "squeezed in" at the expense of others, and it is recommended to have *expanded hours* so that patients with inflexible schedules will be able to come in. Attention should also be placed on making sure that a private physician visit is available when needed, but that other options are available when not. For example, routine visits may be assigned to midlevel practitioners or registered nurses, and group visits for those with similar chronic conditions may be helpful both for patients and for increasing provider productivity.

Role of the Care Manager   The medical home's focus on the patient in care coordination continues after the visit itself. Following it, the patient's care manager should be available to make sure the patient understands her provider's instructions. The care manager also helps the patient locate and choose specialists and other health services. The care manager must inform specialists of any necessary accommodations and share all applicable information, including the patient care plan, and provide the patient with all relevant information as well. Once the patient goes to this other visit, the care manager will follow up and make sure that the PCMH receives all relevant information. This will allow a smooth transition both away from and back to the medical home. It also ensures that the patient is always treated by her health providers with as full an understanding of her health as possible, and that there are no duplicate or unnecessary tests run. The care manager will then take the information obtained from the patient's outside visits and integrate that information into her care plan.

Continuous Quality Improvement   Once care coordination is initially established within a PCMH, it is important to focus on continuous quality improvement. This may include regular meetings of the care team (outside of the daily huddle) to discuss problems and ideas, as well as meetings with patients and their family members to get their feedback as well. Through focusing on how to best improve care coordination by putting the patient at the center of care in discussion and education, the PCMH will allow its providers to practice at the best of their abilities, and it will be a home to healthier and happier patients.

CONCLUSION: PLANETREE DESIGNATION PROMOTES AN INTEGRATED APPROACH TO PATIENT-CENTERED CARE

Though the Patient-Centered Hospital and Resident-Centered Community Designation Program (www.planetree.org) recognizes excellence in patient-centered care at the site level, many of the criteria promote creation of and participation in a patient-centered continuum of care. Specific criteria explicitly address the role of a patient-centered provider in supporting coordinated transitions of care through provision of meaningful discharge and transition instructions, development of processes to support patients in managing their own health information, and cultivation of partnerships with other local health care providers to improve cross-site coordination, communication, and information exchanges (Planetree Inc., 2012).

Other criteria that focus on activating the patient and their informal caregivers to manage their health and wellness further emphasize that patient-centered care is less about the setting where care is provided and more about the person at the center of the care experience. Therefore, pursuing recognition as a Patient-Centered Hospital or Resident-Centered Community is not only a strategy for shoring up an individual establishment's patient-centered culture, but can also be a starting point for the work of creating a full continuum of coordinated, personalized, humanized, and demystified care for a collective population.

REFERENCES

Harman, J. S., Scholle, S. H., Ng, J. H., Pawlson, L. G., and others. "Association of Health Plans' Healthcare Effectiveness Data and Information Set (HEDIS) Performance with Outcomes of Enrollees with Diabetes." *Medical Care*, 2010, *48*, 217–223.

Meyers, D., Peikes, D., Genevro, J., Peterson, and others. "The Roles of Patient-Centered Medical Homes and Accountable Care Organizations in Coordinating Patient Care." Rockville, MD: Agency for Healthcare Research and Quality, Dec. 2010.

Planetree, Inc. "Advancing Person-Centered Care Across the Continuum of Care." *Long-Term Living Magazine*. Accessed Aug. 2012 at www.ltlmagazine.com/ whitepaper/advancing-person-centered-care-across-continuum

Schoen, C., Osborn, R., Squires, D., Doty, M., and others. "New 2011 Survey of Patients with Complex Care Needs in Eleven Countries Finds That Care Is Often Poorly Coordinated." *Health Affairs (Millwood)*, 2011, *30*(12):2437–48

Steele, G. D., Haynes, J. A., Davis, D. E., Tomcavage, J., and others. "How Geisinger's Advanced Medical Home Model Argues the Case for Rapid-Cycle Innovations." *Health Affairs*, 2010, *29*, 2047–2053.

INDEX